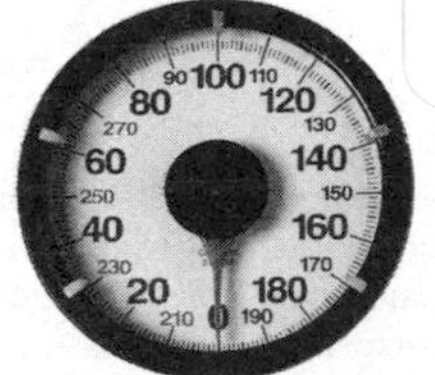

Outwit your Weight JOURNAL

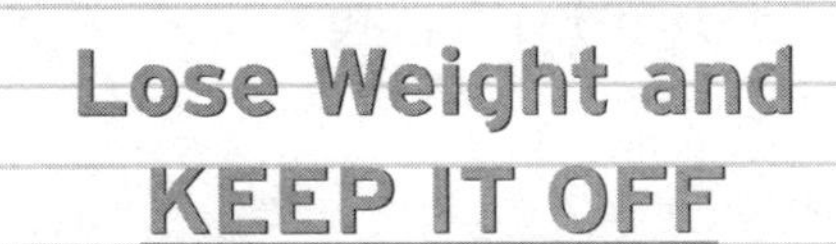

Lose Weight and KEEP IT OFF with This Personalized Weight-Loss Diary

By CATHY NONAS, R.D.
Director, VanItallie Center for Nutrition and Weight Management
at St. Luke's–Roosevelt Hospital

with **Jennifer Bright and Julia VanTine**

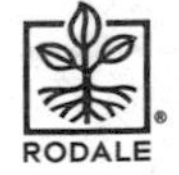

Notice
This book is intended as a reference volume only, not as a medical manual. The information given here is designed to help you make informed decisions about your health. It is not intended as a substitute for any treatment that may have been prescribed by your doctor. If you suspect that you have a medical problem, we urge you to seek competent medical help.

Printed in the United States of America
Rodale Inc. makes every effort to use acid-free ♾, recycled paper ♻.

The calorie burn chart on page 188 is reprinted with permission from Barbara Ainsworth, Ph.D., of the exercise science department at the University of South Carolina in Columbia.

Interior and cover design by Carol Angstadt

Photograph of pen by Andrew Cameron
Photograph of scale by EyeWire Collection

ISBN 1–57954–483–5 paperback

Distributed to the book trade by St. Martin's Press

2 4 6 8 10 9 7 5 3 1 paperback

CONTENTS

INTRODUCTION

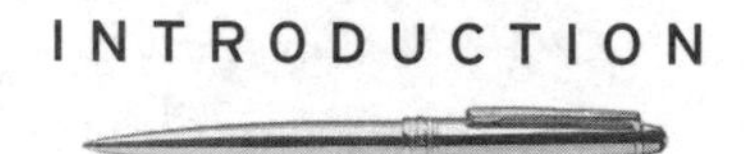

THE ULTIMATE WEIGHT-CONTROL TOOL: A PEN

It will take you just minutes to open this journal each day and jot down what you eat. But this tiny time investment you're about to make will pay off, in pounds off.

Ask Joan. Just 1 week into keeping her food journal, she made an astounding discovery: She was consuming 400 more calories a day than she thought!

She was even more astounded when she did the math. Those 400 extra calories a day added up to 146,000 extra calories a year—the equivalent of 42 pounds!

She made a conscious effort to trim the extra 2,800 calories a week from her diet. And, as a result, she began to peel the extra pounds from her frame.

If, like Joan, you commit to recording in your journal each day every last nibble, taste, and bite, you'll discover, as she did, the eating patterns and pitfalls that sabotage your diet—and your weight.

You nibbled a few cheese and sausage samples at the supermarket deli counter? Consult a calorie counter and you're likely to find that you ingested a couple of hundred calories. You stole "just a few" fries from a friend's plate? Tack on another 100 or so calories.

As you keep your journal, you'll undoubtedly also discover the importance of portion sizes. How many ounces does your cereal bowl hold? Two? Three? More? If you fill your bowl to the brim, you're eating hundreds of calories more than you think, because one serving of cereal is just *1 ounce*. When you keep a journal, lightbulb after lightbulb will go on as you begin to see—in black and white—why you're having trouble losing weight or keeping it off.

You'll also learn more about high-risk situations, how moods affect your eating behavior, and how a rainy day can result in twice as many trips to the kitchen.

Still not convinced? Study after study suggests that people who keep food journals not only lose more weight but also tend to keep those lost pounds lost.

One study found that people gained 500 percent more weight per week during the high-risk holiday season than during non-holiday weeks. But a few actually *lost* weight during the mega-calorie holiday season. Which ones? Those who kept food journals.

In another study, a group that kept detailed food journals for 15 weeks lost 64 percent more weight than those who didn't.

But perhaps the most compelling evidence for food journals comes from the National Weight Control Registry, a group of nearly 3,000 men and women who have lost at least 30 pounds and kept them off for at least a year. Researchers who track these folks and their weight have found that they share many common behaviors, including keeping food journals.

But enough with the science. This food journal *can* help you shed the pounds you've been struggling to lose, maybe for years. Record your food intake every single day, be honest with yourself about what and how much you eat, and you will:

- Discover how, when, and where you consume extra calories.
- Identify specific pitfalls that may be preventing you from making healthy, lasting changes in your eating habits.

- Identify trends, such as eating more during the weekends or gradually reducing your workouts from four times a week to one.
- Become more aware of serving sizes, so you'll eat less.
- Prevent yourself from eating on autopilot by becoming more aware of the food you consume.
- Spot minor slips in your eating habits before they become major derailments.

While this journal can be used alone, it was designed to be used in combination with the book *Outwit Your Weight*. The book includes even more tips, tools, and techniques for weight management.

Most important, though, keeping this journal can help free a previously untapped source of motivation deep within you—a strength and determination you may not have known that you had. As you chart your progress and actually *see* positive change, you'll be more motivated than ever to reach your ultimate goal: a healthier, happier, fitter you.

Don't lose another second.
Let's get started!

Part 1

HOW TO USE THE JOURNALS

WHAT ARE *YOUR* DIET DANGER ZONES?

You "taste" while you cook or bake.

You eat healthfully at home but pig out when you dine out.

Your "cravings" are more like an addiction—when your favorite food whispers your name, you must heed its call.

Situations like these, and many others, are the death of your weight-loss efforts, over and over again.

You're not alone. We *all* have weight-loss weaknesses—specific situations or events that can derail our weight-control efforts and undermine our good intentions.

We call these situations Diet Danger Zones. And if we don't confront them, chances are good that we'll never get off the weight-loss merry-go-round. We'll start diet after diet . . . and even if we lose the weight, we're likely to gain it back because we haven't learned what trips us up. That is, we haven't learned to spot—and defend against—our unique Diet Danger Zones.

If you're determined to lose weight and *keep it off*, you must accomplish two goals. First, you must identify your Diet Danger Zones. Then you have to learn and use tools to defend yourself against them. (More about tools later.) Once you know what stresses and situations drive you toward the Krispy Kremes or Doritos, you'll be able to prepare for them, thereby short-circuiting their destructive power.

Of course, we may never completely eradicate our Diet Danger Zones. (It's not likely, for example, that we'll ever become indifferent to chocolate!) But we *can* learn how to keep them from blindsiding our weight-loss efforts time and again.

There are as many Diet Danger Zones as there are dieters. But 40 come up again and again, and they're listed below. Scan them and zero in on those that speak to you. Throughout this journal, you'll discover unique tips, tools, and techniques to overcome them—ways to help you plan and control your intake of calories, change self-destructive behaviors, become more active, or help you think more positively about yourself, your body, and your weight.

Here's our "top 40 countdown." Which danger zones trip *you* up?

1. You're tired.
2. You're angry.
3. You're bored.
4. You're stressed.
5. You're coping with a major stressor such as a career change, caring for an aging parent, or separation or divorce.
6. You have a craving.
7. You feel a binge coming on.
8. After your workout, you raid the refrigerator.
9. Your job requires you to eat on the run.
10. You're facing a business lunch or dinner.
11. You work at home . . . and the refrigerator beckons.
12. The holiday season has begun.
13. There's a food pusher in your life.
14. Your partner says he "likes you just the way you are."
15. You eat as you cook . . . and then again at the table.
16. You're at a big celebration . . . and when you're happy, you eat.
17. You eat when you read or watch television.
18. You're on a medication that stimulates your appetite.
19. You've been "good," but the scale says you've gained 2 pounds.
20. You've been on a plateau for 2 weeks now.

21. You're on vacation and can't resist the local fare.
22. Your family won't eat healthy fare, and you can't resist their goodies.
23. You're newly in love . . . and you're truly eating for two.
24. You're so bored with your diet that you're ready to hold up a Hostess delivery truck.
25. You've fallen off your exercise plan, which makes you less careful about your diet.
26. You love to cook . . . and want desperately to bake your legendary death by chocolate cake.
27. You're a mall eater.
28. You have Garbage Pail Syndrome . . . you eat the leftovers off your kids' plates.
29. You follow a low-fat diet and eat only low-fat snack foods, but you're gaining weight.
30. You can't get through a movie without an extra-large popcorn.
31. From November 1 to March 31, your willpower goes south with the geese.
32. You're from a culture where food is equated with love.
33. Ever since you stopped smoking, you can't stop eating.
34. Your colleagues bring doughnuts to work.
35. You're a chocolate addict.
36. You get pregnant and gain 15 pounds in the first trimester.
37. You hit menopause and gain 15 pounds overnight.
38. You stick to your diet Monday through Friday afternoon . . . and blow it over the weekend.
39. You skip breakfast and lunch, then inhale the contents of the refrigerator at dinner.
40. You have a diet "supervisor."

TOOLS: YOUR BEST DANGER ZONES DEFENSE

A plumber without a set of wrenches is useless. A hairstylist can't work without scissors.

And a dieter without tools is just as stuck.

If your "job" is to lose weight and keep it off, you need tools that can help you get the job done. Thankfully, you're about to get them.

Simply put, a tool is an action that helps keep you from overeating when you're faced with one of your Diet Danger Zones. It can be as basic as consciously eating more slowly or as ingenious as using chopsticks or a shrimp fork to reinforce the eat-slow message. Tools can help us eat less, move more, and come to view ourselves, our weight, and food in healthier ways.

There are hundreds of tools in this journal and in the companion book. They all fall neatly into four categories: Food Tools, Mood Tools, Move Tools, and Behavior Tools. You might think of these categories as the Four Tool Groups.

Remember learning about the Four Food Groups back in elementary school? The concept was: Eat from all four groups (meat, dairy, grains, and fruits and veggies) and you'll be eating a balanced diet. (FYI: The Basic Four morphed into the Food Guide Pyramid in 1992.)

If you use tools from all four groups, you'll be following a balanced weight-loss program. That's because they'll help you with all of the major components of weight-control success: your food selection and portions, your level of physical activity, your emotional relationship with food, and how you choose to act in the face of temptation.

To introduce you to the Four Tool Groups, read the mini-profile for each group below.

Food Tools

These tools help you manage your intake of calories and nutrients such as fats, carbohydrates, fiber, and protein. Many of these tools will automatically help you follow a low-fat, high-fiber diet. But you'll also find tools that will help you follow virtually any diet plan.

SAMPLE FOOD TOOL: Add air to your menu. Foods like broccoli, lettuce, air-popped popcorn, puffed cereals, and tubular pasta take up a lot of space in your stomach. Making your food look "bigger" helps satisfy your desire for hearty portions.

Mood Tools

While food tools focus primarily on your physical self, mood tools are designed to reshape negative thoughts about yourself and your body into more positive ones. When your thoughts support your weight-loss efforts, it becomes easier—and much more pleasant—to follow a diet and exercise program.

SAMPLE MOOD TOOL: Take a Zen-minute break. At least once a day, find the time to just . . . be. Even 10 to 15 minutes of quiet time per day helps eliminate the white noise in your brain. (Even just 3 minutes twice a day can help!) If you're in the office, close the door and take the phone off the hook. At home, escape to the garden or take your pooch for a quick jaunt around the block.

Move Tools

We all have different levels of physical ability, depending on our current weight and health. But no matter what level you're at, the move tools will help you become more active, both in your everyday life and in sticking to an exercise program.

SAMPLE MOVE TOOL: Become an alley cat. Even if you hate to exercise, it's almost impossible to hate the sport that Ralph Kramden loved: bowling! So go alone, take the kids, or join a league. You'll burn about three times as many calories bowling as you would watching a movie—even if you throw nothing but gutter balls.

Behavior Tools

The aim of behavior tools is to change your behaviors—specifically, self-defeating habits that, unknown to you, are sabotaging your weight-control program. These behaviors include everything from eating in front of the TV to wolfing down your food in 10 minutes flat.

SAMPLE BEHAVIOR TOOL: Avoid popcorn overload. If you tend to snack too much at the movies, start watching the movie without any food. If you must eat, snack on a lollipop from your purse. You'll save calories and money.

JOURNAL DO'S: THE RIGHT WAY TO WRITE DOWN THE POUNDS

Now that you're familiar with the key concepts of this journal—identifying your Diet Danger Zones and using tools to avoid them—you're ready to learn the basics of keeping a food journal.

Don't panic. There's no right or wrong way to keep a journal. The "right" way is *any* way that makes recording your food intake easy—and hopefully fun—to do.

Still, if you've never kept a journal or have been unsuccessful at keeping one in the past, the guidelines below can help.

As you'll see in the next section, there are several ways to use this journal, depending on your weight-loss personality profile. But regardless of which profile you choose, consider starting with the Calorie-Counting Journal and using it for at least 2 weeks before you switch over. (You'll find the how-tos on page 30.) This, the meat and potatoes of food journals, will help you quantify exactly what and how much you're eating. It will also give you a "baseline" from which to measure your progress.

IT'S BEST TO RECORD YOUR FOOD INTAKE EVERY DAY. But if you find you're not up to the task yet, keep your journal for a minimum of 2 weekdays and 1 weekend day a week so that you can chart your progress. Look for trends, such as increased eating on weekend days or lack of physical activity on weekdays.

RECORD WHAT YOU EAT AS SOON AS YOU EAT IT. It's easy to "forget" to record certain foods if you wait until the end of the day to journal.

MEASURE PORTION SIZES OR AT LEAST GUESSTIMATE THEM. When you aren't aware of the size of the serving, you're probably eating larger portions than you realize. For example, there's a significant calorie difference between ½ cup and 1 cup of pasta.

BE HONEST. If you "forget" to record those seven mini chocolate bars you had in a colleague's office or the french fries from your kid's Happy Meal, the only person you're cheating is yourself. And you learn nothing to help you out the next time.

MAKE AN ENTRY EACH TIME YOU EAT. No matter how small the amount, bites and tastes really add up.

Since weekdays are generally more structured than weekends, consider beginning your journal on a weekday. A Monday may be the typical day to start. But any day is the right time to begin.

USE ANY ONE OF THESE JOURNALS FOR AS LONG AS YOU'D LIKE. But if you get bored, switch! The challenge of jumping from journal to journal may make it more fun to continue, and you'll also get to focus on different aspects of your unique eating patterns and behavior. Of course, if you prefer to stick with one kind of journal, that's fine, too.

FIND YOUR WEIGHT-LOSS PERSONALITY PROFILE

Many food journals on the market have you fill out the same information day after day, week after week, month after month. There's nothing wrong with this approach, if it works for you. The fact is, for many of us, filling out the same blank page each day can get mighty dull.

That's why there is a variety of ways to keep this journal—six, to be exact. Use one. Use them all.

Or let us do the work. Read the weight-loss personality profiles below, then select the one that you feel best describes you. In the next section, we'll tell you which of the six journals may be your best "fit." Here are the profiles:

The Baby

MAIN CHARACTERISTIC: Not taking responsibility for what and how much she eats.

FAVORITE QUOTE: "Everyone else can eat it. I want it, too! I want what I want when I want it!"

FREQUENTLY SEEN: Stomping feet and flailing fists.

MINI-PROFILE: Sometimes consciously, sometimes not, Babies believe that they should be able to eat like "everyone else." Or they believe that they're serving others' needs rather than their own when they accept others' invitations or exhortations to eat. Their behavior can masquerade as politeness. For example, at a family gathering, a Baby may think, "My Aunt Lucy went to all this trouble to prepare my favorite—lasagna. How could I be so rude as to turn down seconds?" While Babies can reel off everything they *haven't* eaten, they "forget" what they *have* eaten.

The Ostrich

MAIN CHARACTERISTIC: Denial and magical thinking.
FAVORITE QUOTE: "I didn't eat all *that*." Variations: "I didn't/don't eat that much" or "I'll start my diet tomorrow."
FREQUENTLY SEEN: Shrugging shoulders and looking surprised. Avoiding the scale, believing that if they don't *see* their weight, they won't *be* their weight.
MINI-PROFILE: Ostriches hide what they eat from others—and from themselves. They figure that if no one sees them eat it, then they haven't, in fact, eaten it. And if they "forget" that they've eaten a package of cookies in the car, then those calories can't be absorbed. Ostriches' lack of short-term food memory makes it difficult for them to keep food diaries. What's more, they devise intricate rules about what does and does not "count" when it comes to food. The phrase "It doesn't count if . . ." is an Ostrich catchphrase, as in, "It doesn't count if I eat in the car . . . off someone else's plate . . . out of the container. . . ."

The Restrained Eater

MAIN CHARACTERISTIC: Extremes of dieting and overeating.
FAVORITE QUOTE: "I'll just have one."
FREQUENTLY SEEN: Wearing a pious expression.
MINI-PROFILE: Restrained Eaters eat like birds in public, making everyone wonder, "How in the world can she eat like that and still be so heavy?" The answer: They're always on diets—often, a fly-by-night one—and their constant deprivation leads them to episodes of extreme overeating. When Restrained Eaters go off their plans, they do it in a big way. After all, they're going to start their diets tomorrow.

Restrained Eaters also tend to overeat on "diet" foods such as fat-free cheese or rice cakes. It's possible to eat a block of fat-free cheese and an entire box of fat-free crackers, a smidgen at a time.

The Slow Gainer

MAIN CHARACTERISTIC: Avoidance and poor impulse control.
FAVORITE QUOTE: "I'm gaining half a pound a week, sometimes a couple of pounds in a month! I don't know how it happens. I don't eat that much."
FREQUENTLY SEEN: Stepping on the scale with optimism, then stepping off in shock.
MINI-PROFILE: Many Slow Gainers' destructive eating behaviors are subtle—so subtle that to detect them would require some heavy food-diary analysis. Unfortunately, Slow Gainers rarely keep food diaries. And even if they did, they would probably neglect to write down everything that they put into their mouths—which is unfortunate, because Slow Gainers are slaves to food availability and their own impulses. They may decide to have a salad with blue cheese dressing because they haven't had it in so long or choose the garlic mashed potatoes because they "never" do. They may also bake brownies or another high-calorie treat for the rest of the family and taste while they bake. Slow Gainers often feel victimized because they truly believe that they're doing everything they can to keep their weight down and that they should be rewarded, not punished.

The Weekend Eater

MAIN CHARACTERISTIC: Extremes of vigilance and abandon.
FAVORITE QUOTE: "I eat well and exercise all week. But the weekend is my time for me!"
FREQUENTLY SEEN: Ordering salads and fruit cups Monday through Thursday and the mozzarella appetizers or spicy chicken wings with blue cheese dressing on Friday—and maybe even Saturday and Sunday.
MINI-PROFILE: Weekend Eaters restrict their eating during the week, but once Friday night rolls around, watch out! These folks usually reserve their weekends for socializing and partying, and they can't enjoy themselves if they must monitor their alcohol intake, crunch calories during their Saturday dinner out, or not sample what they make during their Sunday afternoon cooking fest. But like those of

us who don't balance the checkbook, Weekend Eaters end up paying the price—in extra pounds. It's hard to bank all your calories to "spend" on the weekend, and it's even more difficult to make up during the week for letting loose on the weekends.

The Good Fairy/Bad Fairy

MAIN CHARACTERISTIC: Using food as both a reward and a punishment.

FAVORITE QUOTE: "I've been so good. I never eat ice cream, so today I can have some."

FREQUENTLY SEEN: Dutifully ignoring the cheesecake on a friend's kitchen counter, then cruising the bakery section of the supermarket for a slice. Or two.

MINI-PROFILE: To Good Fairies/Bad Fairies, food is a double-edged sword. They view it as both a reward for a job well-done and as a punishment when they feel ashamed and guilty about overeating and its consequences. There's an inherent catch-22 in being a Good Fairy/Bad Fairy. If you've been "good," you deserve the treat. But once you have it, you have to be punished for eating it. Punishment may include starving the next day or even quitting a weight-loss plan.

The Stress Eater

MAIN CHARACTERISTIC: Anxiety, stress, or fear.

FAVORITE QUOTE: Stress Eaters rarely talk. They eat.

FREQUENTLY SEEN: Zoning out in front of the television with a family-size bag of chips.

MINI-PROFILE: To one degree or another, all of us are stress eaters who use food as a tranquilizer. Who hasn't turned to comforting, creamy ice cream or soft, velvety cheesecake to quell the tension caused by long work hours, demanding partners and children, endless bills, and a lack of downtime? (And if our favorite comfort foods aren't available, Jell-O—in powder form—or a few heaping tablespoons of peanut butter work just as well.) But while some people can exorcise stress by going for a walk, soaking in a bubble bath, or crawling into bed to read a few pages of a novel, Stress Eaters tend to turn to food *first* in an effort to anesthetize scary feelings.

CHOOSING THE BEST JOURNAL FOR *YOU*

Now that you've chosen your weight-loss personality profile, you're ready to select the journal that corresponds to your type. Listed beneath each journal type, you'll find the matching personality types. Bear in mind, however, that you should use the journal that most appeals to you, regardless of your profile. Also, consider beginning with the Calorie-Counting Journal.

JOURNAL #1

The Calorie-Counting Journal

For Babies; Ostriches; Good Fairies/Bad Fairies

This no-nonsense journal will likely be most helpful to Good Fairy/Bad Fairy types, who like order and structure, or to Ostriches, who need to get real about how much they're eating. But its appeal also extends to those of us who love numbers. Toting up the calories in each meal and snack and arriving at the grand total at the end of the day can be extremely reassuring and satisfying.

You'll find more detailed instructions, a sample completed page, and a month's worth of blank pages beginning on page 32.

JOURNAL #2

The Food-Mood Journal

For Babies; Stress Eaters; Good Fairies/Bad Fairies

If you typically use food to mute anger, sadness, anxiety, or stress, this journal may be the one for you. Recording not only what you ate but also how you felt as you ate it can help you analyze your episodes of emotional eating, thereby weakening the powerful link between feelings and food. Babies may see a pattern begin to emerge: They may eat out of "duty" because someone prepared their favorite meal, or they may feel sulky because they don't want to miss the fun of after-work drinks and wings with colleagues.

You'll find more detailed instructions, a sample completed page, and a month's worth of blank pages beginning on page 70.

JOURNAL #3

The Portion-Control Journal

For all types, particularly Ostriches

Experts say that, each day, you should eat six to eight servings of grains (breads, cereals, rice, and pasta); at least five servings of fruits and vegetables; two to three servings of high-calcium foods (fat-free milk, fat-free or low-fat yogurt, fat-free or low-fat cheeses, soy milk, and tofu); two to four servings of lean meat, fish, poultry, and eggs; one to two servings of legumes, nuts, and seeds; and 2 tablespoons of monounsaturated fat such as olive oil.

Wow! That's a lot of food. A lot of *healthy* food! In fact, if you actually followed these recommendations, you'd be too full for junk food. To use this journal, find out how many servings of each category you should eat a day, based on your weight. Then check off the boxes that correspond to each category. Finally, record the junk food—if you were actually able to fit some into your stomach.

You'll find more detailed instructions, a sample completed page, and a month's worth of blank pages beginning on page 108.

JOURNAL #4

The Overeating Journal

For Babies; Restrained Eaters

If you are most like the Baby profile, chances are that you're a fairly controlled eater who occasionally (or frequently) "loses it." In this journal, you record *only* those times when you feel you've overeaten or your eating got out of control. You might have 3 such times in a week or 10 in one day. Or you might run into trouble only on weekends.

Just knowing that your journal is with you may discourage you from impulsive overeating. It can also help you see a destructive pattern that's easier to change than you realized.

Page 148 has more detailed instructions, a sample completed page, and a sample blank page to photocopy.

JOURNAL #5

The Social-Butterfly Journal

For Weekend Eaters; Slow Gainers

For some people, the only time they really overeat is in social settings. In this journal, you record what you consume in restaurants, parties, business meals—in real time. For example, if you have three slices of garlic bread, you'd go to the restroom and jot down each slice. (You can also record in public, if it's appropriate.) The goal is to become more aware of how much you consume in social settings.

Page 150 has more detailed instructions, a sample completed page, and a sample blank page to photocopy.

JOURNAL #6

The Fullness Journal

For all types, especially Slow Gainers

For some of us, there's no such thing as being a "little" full. By the time we feel full, we're in actual physical discomfort. If this sounds like you, try this journal.

This journal consists of just three columns: "Stuffed," "Too Full," and "Comfortable." Fill them out every few months to help you become more aware of your own physical symptoms of fullness.

Page 153 has more detailed instructions, a sample completed page, and a sample blank page to photocopy.

SMART STRATEGIES TO USE WITH ANY JOURNAL

No matter which journal you select, the tactics below can help you overcome two common—and stubborn—dangers to any diet: overeating alone and overeating while performing another activity.

The Come-out-of-the-Closet Tactic

For all types, especially Restrained Eaters and Ostriches

If you typically overeat alone, away from the judging eyes of others, use the journal of your choice to record what you eat only when you're alone. Imagine your journal as a caring, nonjudgmental friend. You might write, "I'm about to eat an entire box of glazed doughnuts." Chances are that simply admitting what you're about to do will deflate your urge to actually do it.

The Hand-to-Mouth Tactic

For all types, especially Slow Gainers

If you can't read, surf the Net, or watch your favorite sitcom without a snack, this tactic can help you become aware of "hand-to-mouth behavior." (So named because it's the act of moving the hand to the mouth—not the food itself—that's important.) Simply keep the journal of your choice next to your latest novel or the computer mouse or on top of your TV. When you suddenly realize that you're engaged in mindless eating, you can choose to continue eating, opt for a lower-calorie snack, or stop eating altogether.

GET READY, GET SET, GOAL!

If you're an old hand at the weight-loss game, chances are you've set goals to help you stay on course. Perhaps you've set them more than once, only to fail to attain them and to abandon them altogether.

If this sounds like you, give goals one more shot. The key is to set *realistic* goals—those that provide inspiration as well as a road map to success.

Goals give shape to a dream—in this case, your dream of losing weight for good. They focus your thinking, generate the energy to drive you, and help you stick to the cornerstones of successful weight loss: deliberate planning and determined follow-through.

Still, setting a helpful goal requires thought: "I want to lose 15 pounds" just doesn't cut it. Fortunately, using a few simple guidelines can turn you into an expert goal setter—and increase your odds of success.

So before you sit down to write your goals, read the tips below. As you write, ponder this saying: "An obstacle is something you see when you take your eyes off the goal."

GET LOST IN THE DETAILS. As you formulate your goals, be as specific as you can. The more hows, whens, and whats your goals contain, the clearer your path to success becomes.

Here's an example of a specific goal: "I will consume between 1,300 and 1,600 calories a day [or whatever your calorie allotment is, based on your height and weight] and walk in the park after work on Mondays, Wednesdays, and Fridays for at least 30 minutes." That's a lot different than: "I will eat right and exercise three times a week." Be even more specific by adding "keep sneakers at work, eat nothing after 8:00 P.M., drink a lot of water, eat five servings of vegetables a day," and so on.

SET "NOW" AND "LATER" GOALS. Short-term goals are those that you can attain in weeks or months. Meeting short-term goals allows you to mark your progress—and celebrate it—along the way. One example of a short-term goal might be: "I will aim to eat two vegetables at dinner and fruit at lunch each day for the next 2 months to help boost my nutrient intake."

Meeting short-term goals also sparks your determination to meet your long-term goals, which take 6 months or more to achieve. A long-term goal might be: "I will lose 5 to 10 percent of my weight in 6 months." Losing even a small amount of weight will help lower your risk of developing diseases associated with obesity, such as high blood pressure, diabetes, heart disease, stroke, and certain cancers.

GET REAL. In a perfect world, you could revamp your diet, work out for an hour a day, think positive thoughts constantly, and lose 5 pounds a week. Alas, we don't live on that planet. So give your goals another read to ensure you can actually meet them, given your current fitness level, age, and body type.

ACCENTUATE THE POSITIVE. Word your goals in positive language. Notice the difference between "I will never eat chocolate again" and "Before I eat chocolate, I will eat eight servings of fruits and vegetables each day. If I still crave chocolate, I will treat myself to a miniature chocolate bar—and savor it."

PLAN BUILT-IN REWARDS. Before you even start working toward your first short-term goal, decide how you will reward yourself (with a nonfood reward) once you've met it. (A new hardcover bestseller? A salon manicure or facial?) Reward yourself *big* when you meet a long-term goal—whatever you choose, you've earned it!

TAKE REGULAR "GOAL TESTS." Every time you make a decision that impacts your program during the day, ask yourself, "Does what I'm about to do—or not do—bring me closer to or farther from my goals?" If your answer is "closer to," such as going for a walk with a friend, great. If the answer is "farther from," such as eating out of that ice cream container, well, you know what to do.

BET ON YOUR GOALS. Set goals with a friend who's also trying to lose weight and wager something small—a massage or a bouquet of flowers, for example—on which one of you will achieve her goal first. Healthy competition like this can spark your motivation and help you set more challenging goals.

If you'd rather be collaborative than competitive, make a pact. For example, agree that when either of you meets a goal, you'll treat each other to something special like a movie or a day trip. One study found that this type of group goal, when people are counting on each other to succeed, resulted in 78 percent of the groups meeting their goal.

SEEK SUPPORT. Tell trusted friends and family about your goals so they can help you meet them. Surround yourself with people committed to helping themselves and to helping you help yourself. (This might be a group like Weight Watchers or TOPS.) Just as important, do your best to avoid people you know are negative influences on you. (See Diet Danger Zones #13 and #40.)

VISUALIZE SUCCESS. When you feel discouraged, don't give in to negativity. Instead, close your eyes and picture yourself as you will look and feel once you meet your goals. Don't focus on the sacrifices you're making but the strides you've made and can continue to make. Believe that the unveiling of the new and improved you is only a matter of time, and you'll turn that belief into a self-fulfilling prophecy.

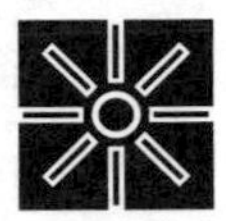

SETTING YOUR GOAL WEIGHT

Now that you know more about how to set realistic and achievable goals, it's time to determine what your goal weight should be. Weight-loss experts use several methods to determine a person's goal weight. Here are two of the simplest.

Body Mass Index

The body mass index (BMI) is a measure of your weight relative to your height. Here's a fairly precise way to calculate your BMI.

1. Multiply your weight in pounds by 0.45 and then round it to the nearest whole number. For example, 150 pounds × 0.45 = 68. This number represents how much you weigh in kilograms.

2. Multiply your height in inches by 0.025. For example, if you're 5 feet 6 inches tall (66 inches), 66 × 0.025 = 1.65, your height in meters.

3. Square the answer from step 2 (1.65 × 1.65) = 2.72.

4. Divide the answer in step 1 by the answer in step 3 (68 ÷ 2.72 = 25). This is your BMI.

If you'd rather not bother with the math, use the chart on the following pages to get a close approximation of your BMI.

BMI	19	20	21	22	23	24	25	26
Height (in.)	**Weight (lb.)**							
58	91	96	100	105	110	115	119	124
59	94	99	104	109	114	119	124	128
60	97	102	107	112	118	123	128	133
61	100	106	111	116	122	127	132	137
62	104	109	115	120	126	131	136	142
63	107	113	118	124	130	135	141	146
64	110	116	122	128	134	140	145	151
65	114	120	126	132	138	144	150	156
66	118	124	130	136	142	148	155	161
67	121	127	134	140	146	153	159	166
68	125	131	138	144	151	158	164	171
69	128	135	142	149	155	162	169	176
70	132	139	146	153	160	167	174	181
71	136	143	150	157	165	172	179	186
72	140	147	154	162	169	177	184	191
73	144	151	159	166	174	182	189	197
74	148	155	163	171	179	186	194	202
75	152	160	168	176	184	191	200	208
76	156	164	172	180	189	197	205	213

To interpret your results, compare your BMI with the ratings below.

<18.5: underweight
18.6–24.9: normal
25–29.9: overweight
>30: obese

Now you can use this information to discover your own personal goal weight.

Say you're 65 inches tall (5 feet 5 inches) and weigh 165 pounds. Your BMI is 27, which puts you in the "overweight" category. If your long-term goal is to get down to the "normal weight" category, you must reduce your BMI to below 25. Check the chart and you'll

27	28	29	30	31	32	33	34	35
129	134	138	143	148	153	158	162	167
133	138	143	148	153	158	163	168	173
138	143	148	153	158	163	168	174	179
143	148	153	158	164	169	174	180	185
147	153	158	164	169	175	180	186	191
152	158	163	169	175	180	186	191	197
157	163	169	174	180	186	192	197	204
162	168	174	180	186	192	198	204	210
167	173	179	186	192	198	204	210	216
172	178	185	191	198	204	211	217	223
177	184	190	197	203	210	216	223	230
182	189	196	203	209	216	223	230	236
188	195	202	209	216	222	229	236	243
193	200	208	215	222	229	236	243	250
199	206	213	221	228	235	242	250	258
204	212	219	227	235	242	250	257	265
210	218	225	233	241	249	256	264	272
216	224	232	240	248	256	264	272	279
221	230	238	246	254	263	271	279	287

see that, at your height, you need to weigh less than 150 pounds to have a BMI of 25. Voilà! So your goal weight could be 149 pounds.

My current weight: ______

My current BMI: ______

My goal weight: ______

My goal BMI: ______

If these numbers seem unrealistic or are overwhelming, even frightening to you, keep in mind that it's true that not everyone will ever get to an ideal BMI. As we've said before, a weight loss of 5 to 10 percent makes you significantly healthier.

Waist Circumference

This measurement is a good indicator of abdominal fat, which in turn is a good indicator of your risk for developing heart disease, high blood pressure, and diabetes. To arrive at your waist circumference, place a measuring tape snugly around your abdomen, right above your hipbone. Disease risk rises if you're a woman with a waist circumference over 35 inches or a man whose waist is over 40 inches.

My current waist circumference: ______

My goal waist circumference: ______

Here's a big-picture look from the National Institutes of Health at how BMI and waist circumference work together.

BMI	DISEASE RISK FOR TYPE 2 DIABETES, HIGH BLOOD PRESSURE, AND HEART DISEASE RELATIVE TO NORMAL WEIGHT AND WAIST CIRCUMFERENCE	
	Men with 40" waist or *less*/ women with 35" waist or *less*	Men with 40" waist or *more*/ women with 35" waist or *more*
<18.5 (underweight)	—	—
18.6–24.9 (normal)	—	—
25–29.9 (overweight)	Increased	High
30–34.9 (obese, class I)	High	Very high
35–39.9 (obese, class II)	Very high	Very high
>40 (extremely obese)	Extremely high	Extremely high

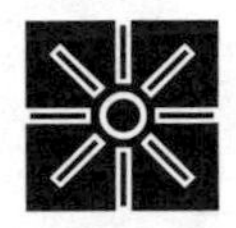

GUIDELINES FOR SETTING DIET AND EXERCISE GOALS

Now that you've determined your long-term weight-loss goal, set similar goals for other components of your program. For example, how many calories and how much fat and fiber should you consume to lose weight safely and effectively? And what's the minimum amount of exercise to strive for? Here are your guidelines.

How many calories? To determine your basal metabolism—the number of calories you burn in a day just to stay alive—multiply your current weight by 10. Then add half of your weight to that number. For example, if you weigh 140 pounds, you burn 1,470 calories each day breathing, pumping blood, and holding your phone to your ear. Add about 400 calories for everyday movement. So you need 1,870 calories to maintain your present weight.

To lose weight, subtract 200 to 500 calories from that number. (The more you subtract, the faster the weight will come off. This will put you in the right range to lose 1 to 2 pounds per week. It's a good idea to talk with your doctor before beginning a diet or exercise program.)

You may be asking: "Why can't I just cut calories instead of increasing exercise plus cutting calories?" You will burn calories, improve your overall health, and tone your body with exercise.

So if you're 140 pounds, you could eat 1,670 calories and burn off 200 calories through exercise.

Now it's time to set your own calorie budget, using the calculations above. (Grab a piece of paper and a pencil or use a calculator: This number-crunching is short and relatively painless.) Once you do, add it to the journal section of the diary on each weekly preview page. (Your calorie goal will change as you lose weight, because you need fewer calories to maintain a lighter weight.)

My daily calorie budget: ______

My daily calorie burn: ______

HOW MUCH EXERCISE? Exercise is more than crucial to weight loss—breaking a sweat on a regular basis may also help you keep those pounds off. The government guideline: moderate exercise for 30 to 45 minutes, 3 to 5 days a week.

My weekly exercise goal: ______

My workout of choice: ______

My calorie burn (see table on page 188): ______

HOW MUCH FAT? Nutrition and weight-loss experts recommend that less than 25 percent of your daily calories come from fat. To arrive at your "fat budget," multiply your daily calorie budget by 0.25. (Here's where your calculator may come in handy.)

If you weigh 140 pounds and choose to subtract 200 calories from your original 1,870, you should aim to consume 1,670 calories each day; no more than 25 percent of them (418 calories) should come from fat. To calculate how many grams of fat you can eat each day, divide the calories in your fat budget by 9. (Each gram of fat contains 9 calories.) In this case, you could eat 46 grams of fat each day. As the number of calories you consume each day goes down, so will the amount of fat.

If you prefer not to count grams of fat, that's fine. Just aim to eat a diet high in naturally low-fat foods like fruits and vegetables.

My daily fat budget (in calories and/or grams): ______

HOW MUCH FIBER? Research suggests that a high-fiber diet can help you not only lose the pounds but also keep them off more easily. In one study, people who ate at least 21 grams of fiber a day gained 8 pounds less over a 10-year period than those who ate less than 12 grams. Other research suggests that a high-fiber diet can reduce your risk of heart disease, cancer, and diabetes. Shoot for 25 to 35 grams of fiber a day.

If you prefer not to count grams of fiber, that's fine, too. Just aim to eat a diet high in naturally high-fiber foods like high-fiber grains, fruits, and vegetables.

My daily fiber goal: ______

If you're following a lower-carbohydrate diet, you may want to count carbohydrates, too. Check the labels for the amount in the foods you buy. Unlike low-fat and high-fiber diets, however, there's little research to support low-carbohydrate diets.

Part 2

THE JOURNALS

SIX JOURNALING STYLES

This is it—you're now ready to start your journal. Get ready to dive in and be prepared to learn more about your eating habits and behaviors than you ever imagined!

In the chapters Find Your Weight-Loss Personality Profile and Choosing the Best Journal for *You*, you selected your profile and chose one of six journals based on that profile. However, we recommend that you begin your journaling journey with the Calorie-Counting Journal, the first journal in this section, and that you use it for at least 2 weeks. The Calorie-Counting Journal is the most traditional of the six, and it asks you to track everything—and we mean everything—you put into your mouth, along with portion sizes. You'll record the calories for each meal and snack and tally up the total at the end of the day.

The Calorie-Counting Journal is a great place to start because it will help you to detect patterns in your eating behaviors. It will also help you develop the self-discipline you need to keep a journal.

After 2 weeks, review your journal with a critical eye. What seem to be your strengths in terms of food choice, time of day, and eating behaviors? Your trouble spots? Do you detect a Diet Danger Zone you didn't think you had? This is the information that will help you sidestep your weight-loss weaknesses and select the tools you need to fight them.

At this point, you can move on to the journal of your choice and switch as often as you like. Some of the journals begin with a week opener page, which you'll fill out at the beginning of each week. Record your beginning weight for the week and the date and the number of days that you've been keeping a journal.

Then read through the weight-loss tools for the week. Each week offers four new tools: a food tool, a mood tool, a move tool, and a behavior tool. Try as many as you can.

Fill in the Danger Zones that you expect to encounter during the week. For example, you may know that you're going to a party Friday night and that your best friend will bring her homemade cheesecake, which you love. Or maybe you're a mall eater, and you have to go there to pick up a baby shower gift. How will you resist the rapturous aroma drifting from the Cinnabon shop? Brainstorm ways to beat those Danger Zones and remember to use your tools.

Next, fill in your goals for the week. You calculated them in Guidelines for Setting Diet and Exercise Goals on page 25. Fill in the number of calories you hope to burn through exercise.

Finally, savor the motivational thought for the week. It's meant to help you through the tough times and cheer you on when you're feeling strong.

Then you can move on to the week's worth of journal pages.

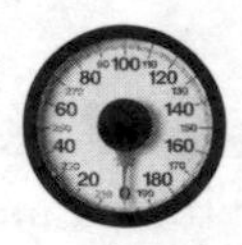

The Calorie-Counting Journal

Here's how to use this journal.

At the top of the page, fill in the date and the number of days you've been keeping the journal.

Then, as you go through your day, record every morsel of food you put into your mouth, along with the portion size. Remember to record snacks and beverages, too. (You may be surprised by how many calories you *drink* each day, especially if you're a soda or fruit-juice junkie.)

There's also room to record the number of calories and grams of fat you consumed at each meal and snack. For example, if your goal is to eat less than 1,270 calories and 35 grams of fat, but by the end of the day you've eaten 1,500 calories and 45 grams of fat, you can see clearly how—and where—you need to adjust your eating.

In the "Happy?" column, record whether you're pleased with the food choice you made. Filling this column in will help you really think about your food choices.

Check off the numbers of servings of water you drink. Aim for at least eight 8-ounce glasses a day.

Check off the number of servings of fruits and vegetables you eat each day. Shoot for nine. See page 108 for a complete description of serving sizes.

Fill in whatever exercise you did. To calculate the number of calories you burned, based on your weight, see the chart on page 188.

At the end of the week, fill out the weekly review page. Repeat the whole process for the following weeks.

DATE *4/5/02* **DAY** *1*

CALORIE-COUNTING JOURNAL

SAMPLE PAGE

Record everything you ate today:

FOOD	CALORIES	FAT	HAPPY?
MORNING			
1½ oz. bran-flakes cereal	*152*	*0.8*	*Yes*
½ cup 1% milk	*51*	*1.3*	*Yes*
1 piece fruit	*81*	*0.5*	*Yes*
MIDDAY			
1 can diet soda	*0*	*0*	*No*
Shrimp cocktail (6 shrimp, ¼ cup sauce)	*65*	*2.5*	*Yes*
2 breadsticks	*50*	*1.2*	*No*
Salad with 2 cups lettuce, 1 cup vegetables	*54*	*0.1*	*No*
2 Tbsp. Italian dressing	*110*	*11*	*Yes*
EVENING			
5 oz. filet mignon	*298*	*14*	*Yes*
1 med. baked potato	*145*	*0.2*	*Yes*
½ Tbsp. butter	*51*	*6*	*No*
½ cup green beans (in butter)	*22*	*0.2*	*No*
1 glass wine	*124*	*0*	*Yes*
SNACKS			
3 small cookies	*147*	*3.1*	*Yes*
1 cup fat-free milk	*86*	*0.4*	*Yes*
1 cup fresh berries	*85*	*0.6*	*Yes*
BITES & TASTES			
1½ pretzels	*35*	*0.3*	*No*
2 bites leftover Chinese food	*28*	*0.7*	*No*
TOTAL:	*1,584*	*42.9*	

If you're following a high-fiber plan, record that amount: Fiber (g)_______

If you're following a lower-carb plan, record that amount: Carbs (g)______

Check off each serving you had of the following:

WATER ☒ ☒ ☒ ☒ ☒ ☒ ☒ ☒ FRUITS & VEGETABLES ☒ ☒ ☒ ☒ ☒ ☒ ☐ ☐ ☐

Exercise completed today: *Walked for 30 minutes* **Calories burned:** *112*

My thoughts and feelings on today's eating and exercise: *Today I feel that I ate a very balanced diet. I was able to choose a healthy meal, even though I ate at a restaurant for dinner.*

WEEK 1

CALORIE-COUNTING JOURNAL

DATE: ______ DAY: ______ WEEK-BEGINNING WEIGHT: ______

WEIGHT-LOSS TOOLS TO TRY THIS WEEK:

FOOD TOOL: Earmark "occasion" foods. For instance, eat hamburgers and hot dogs only at picnics and popcorn only at the movies. This way, you aren't giving up favorites, just saving them for special occasions.

MOOD TOOL: When you feel blue, reach for the phone, a book, or the bubbles (as in a relaxing bath) rather than for a bag of cheese crunchies. These distractions can ward off negative feelings—and the urge to eat. Plus, it's tough to eat in the tub.

MOVE TOOL: Buy a new CD or tape but allow yourself the luxury of listening to it only during your walks or when you are able to dance to it.

BEHAVIOR TOOL: Start a "Take your sneakers to work day" and ask a colleague (or a group of colleagues) if she'd like to walk during lunch. Having comfortable walking shoes with you and making a commitment to a friend can help get you out of the office and to the park or walking path.

Anticipated Diet Danger Zones for this week:

______

Strategies to combat them:

______

______

Goals for the week:

______

______

Daily calorie budget: ______ **Daily fat budget:** ______

Calories to burn each day with exercise: ______

MOTIVATIONAL THOUGHT FOR THE WEEK:

Here's to new beginnings and believing that change is good!

—Cyberdiet.com

DATE ____________ **DAY** ____________

Record everything you ate today:

FOOD	CALORIES	FAT	HAPPY?
MORNING			
MIDDAY			
EVENING			
SNACKS			
BITES & TASTES			
TOTAL:			

If you're following a high-fiber plan, record that amount: Fiber (g)________

If you're following a lower-carb plan, record that amount: Carbs (g)______

Check off each serving you had of the following:

WATER ☐ ☐ ☐ ☐ ☐ ☐ ☐ ☐ FRUITS & VEGETABLES ☐ ☐ ☐ ☐ ☐ ☐ ☐ ☐ ☐

Exercise completed today: ______________________ **Calories burned:** ___

My thoughts and feelings on today's eating and exercise: ____________

____

____

DATE ____________ DAY ____________

Record everything you ate today:

FOOD	CALORIES	FAT	HAPPY?
MORNING			
MIDDAY			
EVENING			
SNACKS			
BITES & TASTES			
TOTAL:			

If you're following a high-fiber plan, record that amount: Fiber (g)________

If you're following a lower-carb plan, record that amount: Carbs (g)______

Check off each serving you had of the following:

WATER ☐ ☐ ☐ ☐ ☐ ☐ ☐ ☐ FRUITS & VEGETABLES ☐ ☐ ☐ ☐ ☐ ☐ ☐ ☐ ☐

Exercise completed today: ______________________ **Calories burned:** ___

My thoughts and feelings on today's eating and exercise: ____________

____

____

DATE ________ **DAY** ________

Record everything you ate today:

FOOD	CALORIES	FAT	HAPPY?
MORNING			
MIDDAY			
EVENING			
SNACKS			
BITES & TASTES			
TOTAL:			

If you're following a high-fiber plan, record that amount: Fiber (g)________

If you're following a lower-carb plan, record that amount: Carbs (g)______

Check off each serving you had of the following:

WATER ☐ ☐ ☐ ☐ ☐ ☐ ☐ ☐ FRUITS & VEGETABLES ☐ ☐ ☐ ☐ ☐ ☐ ☐ ☐ ☐

Exercise completed today: ______________________ **Calories burned:** ___

My thoughts and feelings on today's eating and exercise: ______________

____

____

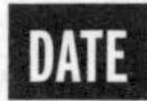

____________ DAY __________

Record everything you ate today:

FOOD	CALORIES	FAT	HAPPY?
MORNING			
MIDDAY			
EVENING			
SNACKS			
BITES & TASTES			
TOTAL:			

If you're following a high-fiber plan, record that amount: Fiber (g)_______

If you're following a lower-carb plan, record that amount: Carbs (g)______

Check off each serving you had of the following:

WATER ☐ ☐ ☐ ☐ ☐ ☐ ☐ ☐ FRUITS & VEGETABLES ☐ ☐ ☐ ☐ ☐ ☐ ☐ ☐ ☐

Exercise completed today: ____________________ **Calories burned:** ___

My thoughts and feelings on today's eating and exercise: ____________

____

____

DATE ____________ **DAY** __________

Record everything you ate today:

FOOD	CALORIES	FAT	HAPPY?
MORNING			
MIDDAY			
EVENING			
SNACKS			
BITES & TASTES			
TOTAL:			

If you're following a high-fiber plan, record that amount: Fiber (g)________

If you're following a lower-carb plan, record that amount: Carbs (g)______

Check off each serving you had of the following:

WATER ☐ ☐ ☐ ☐ ☐ ☐ ☐ ☐ FRUITS & VEGETABLES ☐ ☐ ☐ ☐ ☐ ☐ ☐ ☐ ☐

Exercise completed today: ______________________ **Calories burned:** ___

My thoughts and feelings on today's eating and exercise: _____________

____

____

DATE ____________ 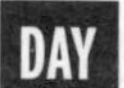 ____________

Record everything you ate today:

FOOD	CALORIES	FAT	HAPPY?
MORNING			
MIDDAY			
EVENING			
SNACKS			
BITES & TASTES			
TOTAL:			

If you're following a high-fiber plan, record that amount: Fiber (g)________

If you're following a lower-carb plan, record that amount: Carbs (g)______

Check off each serving you had of the following:

WATER ☐ ☐ ☐ ☐ ☐ ☐ ☐ ☐ FRUITS & VEGETABLES ☐ ☐ ☐ ☐ ☐ ☐ ☐ ☐ ☐

Exercise completed today: ______________________ **Calories burned:** ___

My thoughts and feelings on today's eating and exercise: _____________

____

____

DATE ____________ 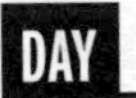 ____________

Record everything you ate today:

FOOD	CALORIES	FAT	HAPPY?
MORNING			
MIDDAY			
EVENING			
SNACKS			
BITES & TASTES			
TOTAL:			

If you're following a high-fiber plan, record that amount: Fiber (g)________

If you're following a lower-carb plan, record that amount: Carbs (g)______

Check off each serving you had of the following:

WATER ☐ ☐ ☐ ☐ ☐ ☐ ☐ ☐ FRUITS & VEGETABLES ☐ ☐ ☐ ☐ ☐ ☐ ☐ ☐ ☐

Exercise completed today: ______________________ **Calories burned:** ___

My thoughts and feelings on today's eating and exercise: _____________

____

____

Weekly Review

DATE: __________ DAY: ________

WEEK-ENDING WEIGHT: ______ WEIGHT CHANGE THIS WEEK: ______

Diet Danger Zones encountered: ________________________________

____

____

____

Most helpful tools used: ____

____

____

____

Least helpful tools used: ____

____

____

____

Patterns I noticed this week: ____________________________________

____

____

____

This week I learned that: ____

____

____

____

How well did I eat this week in relation to my calorie, fat, and fiber budgets? ____

____

____

____

WEEK 2

CALORIE-COUNTING JOURNAL

DATE: ______ DAY: ______ WEEK-BEGINNING WEIGHT: ______

WEIGHT-LOSS TOOLS TO TRY THIS WEEK:

FOOD TOOL: Chunk your salad. Chop rather than shred or slice vegetables. Because it takes more effort to eat bigger pieces, you'll do more chewing and less eating later. Plus, it's less effort to prepare.

MOOD TOOL: When you're lacking motivation, go to your kitchen and spend several minutes carrying a 5-pound bag of sugar. Heavy, right? Do you really want to carry it permanently?

MOVE TOOL: Map a mile. Drive through your neighborhood, using your odometer to find a good 1-mile walking route. While you're at it, map out 1½-, 2-, and 2½-mile routes for days when you're up to a longer workout.

BEHAVIOR TOOL: Pace yourself. Write a note to remind yourself to eat more slowly. Your brain will help you lose weight by letting you know you're satisfied sooner so you stop eating earlier and eat less.

Anticipated Diet Danger Zones for this week:

____

Strategies to combat them:

____

____

Goals for the week:

____

____

Daily calorie budget: ______ **Daily fat budget:** ______

Calories to burn each day with exercise: _____

MOTIVATIONAL THOUGHT FOR THE WEEK:

Never let yourself get too hungry, angry, lonely, or tired.

DATE ____________ 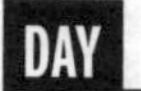 ____________

Record everything you ate today:

FOOD	CALORIES	FAT	HAPPY?
MORNING			
MIDDAY			
EVENING			
SNACKS			
BITES & TASTES			
TOTAL:			

If you're following a high-fiber plan, record that amount: Fiber (g)________

If you're following a lower-carb plan, record that amount: Carbs (g)______

Check off each serving you had of the following:

WATER □ □ □ □ □ □ □ □ FRUITS & VEGETABLES □ □ □ □ □ □ □ □ □

Exercise completed today: ______________________ **Calories burned:** ___

My thoughts and feelings on today's eating and exercise: _____________

____

____

DATE ____________ **DAY** ____________

Record everything you ate today:

FOOD	CALORIES	FAT	HAPPY?
MORNING			
MIDDAY			
EVENING			
SNACKS			
BITES & TASTES			
TOTAL:			

If you're following a high-fiber plan, record that amount: Fiber (g)______

If you're following a lower-carb plan, record that amount: Carbs (g)______

Check off each serving you had of the following:

WATER ☐ ☐ ☐ ☐ ☐ ☐ ☐ ☐ FRUITS & VEGETABLES ☐ ☐ ☐ ☐ ☐ ☐ ☐ ☐ ☐

Exercise completed today: ____________________ **Calories burned:** ___

My thoughts and feelings on today's eating and exercise: ____________

____

____

DATE ____________ 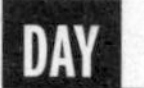 ____________

Record everything you ate today:

FOOD	CALORIES	FAT	HAPPY?
MORNING			
MIDDAY			
EVENING			
SNACKS			
BITES & TASTES			
TOTAL:			

If you're following a high-fiber plan, record that amount: Fiber (g)________

If you're following a lower-carb plan, record that amount: Carbs (g)______

Check off each serving you had of the following:

WATER ☐ ☐ ☐ ☐ ☐ ☐ ☐ ☐ FRUITS & VEGETABLES ☐ ☐ ☐ ☐ ☐ ☐ ☐ ☐ ☐

Exercise completed today: ______________________ **Calories burned:** ___

My thoughts and feelings on today's eating and exercise: _____________

____

____

DATE ____________ **DAY** ____________

Record everything you ate today:

FOOD	CALORIES	FAT	HAPPY?
MORNING			
MIDDAY			
EVENING			
SNACKS			
BITES & TASTES			
TOTAL:			

If you're following a high-fiber plan, record that amount: Fiber (g)_______

If you're following a lower-carb plan, record that amount: Carbs (g)______

Check off each serving you had of the following:

WATER ☐ ☐ ☐ ☐ ☐ ☐ ☐ ☐ FRUITS & VEGETABLES ☐ ☐ ☐ ☐ ☐ ☐ ☐ ☐ ☐

Exercise completed today: ______________________ **Calories burned:** ___

My thoughts and feelings on today's eating and exercise: ____________

____

____

DATE ______ 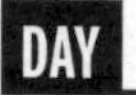 ______

Record everything you ate today:

FOOD	CALORIES	FAT	HAPPY?
MORNING			
MIDDAY			
EVENING			
SNACKS			
BITES & TASTES			
TOTAL:			

If you're following a high-fiber plan, record that amount: Fiber (g)______

If you're following a lower-carb plan, record that amount: Carbs (g)______

Check off each serving you had of the following:

WATER ☐ ☐ ☐ ☐ ☐ ☐ ☐ ☐ FRUITS & VEGETABLES ☐ ☐ ☐ ☐ ☐ ☐ ☐ ☐ ☐

Exercise completed today: ____________________ **Calories burned:** ___

My thoughts and feelings on today's eating and exercise: ____________

____

____

DATE ____________ **DAY** ____________

Record everything you ate today:

FOOD	CALORIES	FAT	HAPPY?
MORNING			
MIDDAY			
EVENING			
SNACKS			
BITES & TASTES			
TOTAL:			

If you're following a high-fiber plan, record that amount: Fiber (g)________

If you're following a lower-carb plan, record that amount: Carbs (g)______

Check off each serving you had of the following:

WATER ☐ ☐ ☐ ☐ ☐ ☐ ☐ ☐ FRUITS & VEGETABLES ☐ ☐ ☐ ☐ ☐ ☐ ☐ ☐ ☐

Exercise completed today: ______________________ **Calories burned:** ___

My thoughts and feelings on today's eating and exercise: ____________

____

____

DATE ____________ **DAY** ____________

Record everything you ate today:

FOOD	CALORIES	FAT	HAPPY?
MORNING			
MIDDAY			
EVENING			
SNACKS			
BITES & TASTES			
TOTAL:			

If you're following a high-fiber plan, record that amount: Fiber (g)_______

If you're following a lower-carb plan, record that amount: Carbs (g)______

Check off each serving you had of the following:

WATER ☐ ☐ ☐ ☐ ☐ ☐ ☐ ☐ FRUITS & VEGETABLES ☐ ☐ ☐ ☐ ☐ ☐ ☐ ☐ ☐

Exercise completed today: ____________________ **Calories burned:** ___

My thoughts and feelings on today's eating and exercise: ____________

____

____

Weekly Review

DATE: ________ DAY: ________

WEEK-ENDING WEIGHT: ______ WEIGHT CHANGE THIS WEEK: ______

Diet Danger Zones encountered: ______________________________

____

____

____

Most helpful tools used: ______________________________

____

____

____

Least helpful tools used: ______________________________

____

____

____

Patterns I noticed this week: ______________________________

____

____

____

This week I learned that: ______________________________

____

____

____

How well did I eat this week in relation to my calorie, fat, and fiber budgets? ______________________________

____

____

____

WEEK 3

CALORIE-COUNTING JOURNAL

DATE: _______ DAY: _______ WEEK-BEGINNING WEIGHT: _______

WEIGHT-LOSS TOOLS TO TRY THIS WEEK:

FOOD TOOL: Fill your plate with two kinds of vegetables. You'll nourish your body with more vitamins and minerals—and you'll have less room on your plate for fattening foods.

MOOD TOOL: Stick inspiring quotes about weight loss or exercise in strategic spots where you might need some extra motivation: on the fridge, TV, car dashboard, or computer.

MOVE TOOL: Count backward. When counting repetitions, such as for situps or steps in a walk, count backward instead of forward—from 10 to 1 instead of 1 to 10. Time will go faster.

BEHAVIOR TOOL: Collect healthy information. As you read books and magazines, clip out or copy inspirational stories, healthy recipes, and informative articles that appeal to you. Gather them in an envelope or three-ring binder. Look at your collection when you need ideas or motivation.

Anticipated Diet Danger Zones for this week:

____

Strategies to combat them:

____

____

Goals for the week:

____

____

Daily calorie budget: ______ **Daily fat budget:** ______

Calories to burn each day with exercise: _____

MOTIVATIONAL THOUGHT FOR THE WEEK:

Don't eat your words. Use them to talk.

—Cathy Nonas, R.D.

DATE ____________ **DAY** ____________

Record everything you ate today:

FOOD	CALORIES	FAT	HAPPY?
MORNING			
MIDDAY			
EVENING			
SNACKS			
BITES & TASTES			
TOTAL:			

If you're following a high-fiber plan, record that amount: Fiber (g)________

If you're following a lower-carb plan, record that amount: Carbs (g)______

Check off each serving you had of the following:

WATER ☐ ☐ ☐ ☐ ☐ ☐ ☐ ☐ FRUITS & VEGETABLES ☐ ☐ ☐ ☐ ☐ ☐ ☐ ☐ ☐

Exercise completed today: ________________________ **Calories burned:** ____

My thoughts and feelings on today's eating and exercise: ______________

____

____

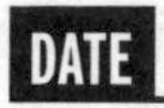
DATE ______

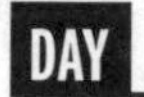
DAY ______

Record everything you ate today:

FOOD	CALORIES	FAT	HAPPY?
MORNING			
MIDDAY			
EVENING			
SNACKS			
BITES & TASTES			
TOTAL:			

If you're following a high-fiber plan, record that amount: Fiber (g)______

If you're following a lower-carb plan, record that amount: Carbs (g)______

Check off each serving you had of the following:

WATER ☐ ☐ ☐ ☐ ☐ ☐ ☐ ☐ FRUITS & VEGETABLES ☐ ☐ ☐ ☐ ☐ ☐ ☐ ☐ ☐

Exercise completed today: ____________________ **Calories burned:** ___

My thoughts and feelings on today's eating and exercise: ____________

____

____

DATE ____________ 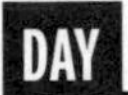 DAY ____________

Record everything you ate today:

FOOD	CALORIES	FAT	HAPPY?
MORNING			
MIDDAY			
EVENING			
SNACKS			
BITES & TASTES			
TOTAL:			

If you're following a high-fiber plan, record that amount: Fiber (g)________

If you're following a lower-carb plan, record that amount: Carbs (g)______

Check off each serving you had of the following:

WATER ☐ ☐ ☐ ☐ ☐ ☐ ☐ ☐ FRUITS & VEGETABLES ☐ ☐ ☐ ☐ ☐ ☐ ☐ ☐ ☐

Exercise completed today: ______________________ Calories burned: ___

My thoughts and feelings on today's eating and exercise: ____________

____

____

DATE ____________ 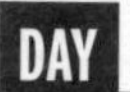 ____________

Record everything you ate today:

FOOD	CALORIES	FAT	HAPPY?
MORNING			
MIDDAY			
EVENING			
SNACKS			
BITES & TASTES			
TOTAL:			

If you're following a high-fiber plan, record that amount: Fiber (g)________

If you're following a lower-carb plan, record that amount: Carbs (g)______

Check off each serving you had of the following:

WATER ☐ ☐ ☐ ☐ ☐ ☐ ☐ ☐ FRUITS & VEGETABLES ☐ ☐ ☐ ☐ ☐ ☐ ☐ ☐ ☐

Exercise completed today: ______________________ **Calories burned:** ___

My thoughts and feelings on today's eating and exercise: _____________

____

____

DATE ____________ **DAY** ____________

Record everything you ate today:

FOOD	CALORIES	FAT	HAPPY?
MORNING			
MIDDAY			
EVENING			
SNACKS			
BITES & TASTES			
TOTAL:			

If you're following a high-fiber plan, record that amount: Fiber (g)________

If you're following a lower-carb plan, record that amount: Carbs (g)______

Check off each serving you had of the following:

WATER ☐ ☐ ☐ ☐ ☐ ☐ ☐ ☐ FRUITS & VEGETABLES ☐ ☐ ☐ ☐ ☐ ☐ ☐ ☐ ☐

Exercise completed today: ______________________ **Calories burned:** ___

My thoughts and feelings on today's eating and exercise: ______________

____

____

DATE ________ 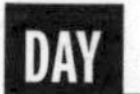 ________

Record everything you ate today:

FOOD	CALORIES	FAT	HAPPY?
MORNING			
MIDDAY			
EVENING			
SNACKS			
BITES & TASTES			
TOTAL:			

If you're following a high-fiber plan, record that amount: Fiber (g)________

If you're following a lower-carb plan, record that amount: Carbs (g)______

Check off each serving you had of the following:

WATER ☐ ☐ ☐ ☐ ☐ ☐ ☐ ☐ FRUITS & VEGETABLES ☐ ☐ ☐ ☐ ☐ ☐ ☐ ☐ ☐

Exercise completed today: ______________________ **Calories burned:** ___

My thoughts and feelings on today's eating and exercise: ______________

____

____

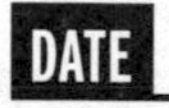 ____________ DAY ____________

Record everything you ate today:

FOOD	CALORIES	FAT	HAPPY?
MORNING			
MIDDAY			
EVENING			
SNACKS			
BITES & TASTES			
TOTAL:			

If you're following a high-fiber plan, record that amount: Fiber (g)________

If you're following a lower-carb plan, record that amount: Carbs (g)______

Check off each serving you had of the following:

WATER ☐ ☐ ☐ ☐ ☐ ☐ ☐ ☐ FRUITS & VEGETABLES ☐ ☐ ☐ ☐ ☐ ☐ ☐ ☐ ☐

Exercise completed today: ______________________ **Calories burned:** ____

My thoughts and feelings on today's eating and exercise: _____________

____

____

Weekly Review

DATE: __________ DAY: _________

WEEK-ENDING WEIGHT: ______ WEIGHT CHANGE THIS WEEK: ______

Diet Danger Zones encountered: ______________________________

____

____

____

Most helpful tools used: ______________________________

____

____

____

Least helpful tools used: ______________________________

____

____

____

Patterns I noticed this week: ______________________________

____

____

____

This week I learned that: ______________________________

____

____

____

How well did I eat this week in relation to my calorie, fat, and fiber budgets? ______________________________

____

____

____

WEEK 4

CALORIE-COUNTING JOURNAL

DATE: _______ DAY: _______ WEEK-BEGINNING WEIGHT: _______

WEIGHT-LOSS TOOLS TO TRY THIS WEEK:

FOOD TOOL: Spoon up chunky soups. In one study, people who ate soup with large vegetable pieces felt fuller and ate 20 percent less during lunch than those who ate pureed soup made with the same ingredients.

MOOD TOOL: Be firm with yourself. Everybody has the same number of hours in a day. Other people—with lives just as busy as yours—find time to do something good for their bodies each day. You can, too. You just have to make it a priority.

MOVE TOOL: Consider your health, then move your butt. Researchers reviewed the medical costs of active folks (specifically, those who exercised moderately or strenuously for at least 30 minutes three or more times a week) compared with those of inactive people. They found that the active people saved $330 in medical expenses a year, such as doctor visits, hospitalization, and medication.

BEHAVIOR TOOL: Brace yourself for this one. If you're in desperate need of motivation, go to the nearest mall. Go to a clothing store and try on something that's one size too small. How much work would you have to do to get into that size? Go for it!

Anticipated Diet Danger Zones for this week:

____

Strategies to combat them:

____

____

Goals for the week:

____

____

Daily calorie budget: ______ **Daily fat budget:** ______

Calories to burn each day with exercise: _____

MOTIVATIONAL THOUGHT FOR THE WEEK:

Think of yourself as a fit and healthy person
who's just temporarily overweight.

—Cyberdiet.com

DATE ____________ **DAY** ____________

Record everything you ate today:

FOOD	CALORIES	FAT	HAPPY?
MORNING			
MIDDAY			
EVENING			
SNACKS			
BITES & TASTES			
TOTAL:			

If you're following a high-fiber plan, record that amount: Fiber (g)________

If you're following a lower-carb plan, record that amount: Carbs (g)______

Check off each serving you had of the following:

WATER ☐ ☐ ☐ ☐ ☐ ☐ ☐ ☐ FRUITS & VEGETABLES ☐ ☐ ☐ ☐ ☐ ☐ ☐ ☐ ☐

Exercise completed today: ______________________ **Calories burned:** ___

My thoughts and feelings on today's eating and exercise: _____________

____

____

DATE ____________ **DAY** ________

Record everything you ate today:

FOOD	CALORIES	FAT	HAPPY?
MORNING			
MIDDAY			
EVENING			
SNACKS			
BITES & TASTES			
TOTAL:			

If you're following a high-fiber plan, record that amount: Fiber (g)________

If you're following a lower-carb plan, record that amount: Carbs (g)______

Check off each serving you had of the following:

WATER ☐ ☐ ☐ ☐ ☐ ☐ ☐ ☐ FRUITS & VEGETABLES ☐ ☐ ☐ ☐ ☐ ☐ ☐ ☐ ☐

Exercise completed today: ______________________ **Calories burned:** ___

My thoughts and feelings on today's eating and exercise: ______________

____

____

DATE ____________ 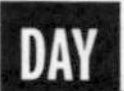 ____________

Record everything you ate today:

FOOD	CALORIES	FAT	HAPPY?
MORNING			
MIDDAY			
EVENING			
SNACKS			
BITES & TASTES			
TOTAL:			

If you're following a high-fiber plan, record that amount: Fiber (g)________

If you're following a lower-carb plan, record that amount: Carbs (g)______

Check off each serving you had of the following:

WATER ☐ ☐ ☐ ☐ ☐ ☐ ☐ ☐ FRUITS & VEGETABLES ☐ ☐ ☐ ☐ ☐ ☐ ☐ ☐ ☐

Exercise completed today: ______________________ **Calories burned:** ___

My thoughts and feelings on today's eating and exercise: ______________

____

____

DATE ____________ DAY ____________

Record everything you ate today:

FOOD	CALORIES	FAT	HAPPY?
MORNING			
MIDDAY			
EVENING			
SNACKS			
BITES & TASTES			
TOTAL:			

If you're following a high-fiber plan, record that amount: Fiber (g)________

If you're following a lower-carb plan, record that amount: Carbs (g)______

Check off each serving you had of the following:

WATER ☐ ☐ ☐ ☐ ☐ ☐ ☐ ☐ FRUITS & VEGETABLES ☐ ☐ ☐ ☐ ☐ ☐ ☐ ☐ ☐

Exercise completed today: ______________________ Calories burned: ___

My thoughts and feelings on today's eating and exercise: ______________

____

____

DATE ____________ 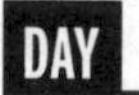

____

Record everything you ate today:

FOOD	CALORIES	FAT	HAPPY?
MORNING			
MIDDAY			
EVENING			
SNACKS			
BITES & TASTES			
TOTAL:			

If you're following a high-fiber plan, record that amount: Fiber (g)________

If you're following a lower-carb plan, record that amount: Carbs (g)______

Check off each serving you had of the following:

WATER ☐ ☐ ☐ ☐ ☐ ☐ ☐ ☐ FRUITS & VEGETABLES ☐ ☐ ☐ ☐ ☐ ☐ ☐ ☐ ☐

Exercise completed today: ______________________ **Calories burned:** ___

My thoughts and feelings on today's eating and exercise: _____________

____

____

DATE ______________ **DAY** ______________

Record everything you ate today:

FOOD	CALORIES	FAT	HAPPY?
MORNING			
MIDDAY			
EVENING			
SNACKS			
BITES & TASTES			
TOTAL:			

If you're following a high-fiber plan, record that amount: Fiber (g)_______

If you're following a lower-carb plan, record that amount: Carbs (g)_____

Check off each serving you had of the following:

WATER ☐ ☐ ☐ ☐ ☐ ☐ ☐ ☐ FRUITS & VEGETABLES ☐ ☐ ☐ ☐ ☐ ☐ ☐ ☐ ☐

Exercise completed today: ____________________ **Calories burned:** ___

My thoughts and feelings on today's eating and exercise: ____________

____

____

DATE ____________ **DAY** ____________

Record everything you ate today:

FOOD	CALORIES	FAT	HAPPY?
MORNING			
MIDDAY			
EVENING			
SNACKS			
BITES & TASTES			
TOTAL:			

If you're following a high-fiber plan, record that amount: Fiber (g)________

If you're following a lower-carb plan, record that amount: Carbs (g)______

Check off each serving you had of the following:

WATER ☐ ☐ ☐ ☐ ☐ ☐ ☐ ☐ FRUITS & VEGETABLES ☐ ☐ ☐ ☐ ☐ ☐ ☐ ☐ ☐

Exercise completed today: ______________________ **Calories burned:** ___

My thoughts and feelings on today's eating and exercise: ______________

____

____

Weekly Review

DATE: __________ DAY: _________

WEEK-ENDING WEIGHT: ______ WEIGHT CHANGE THIS WEEK: ______

Diet Danger Zones encountered: ________________________________

____

____

____

Most helpful tools used: ____________________________________

____

____

____

Least helpful tools used: ___________________________________

____

____

____

Patterns I noticed this week: ________________________________

____

____

____

This week I learned that: ___________________________________

____

____

____

How well did I eat this week in relation to my calorie, fat, and fiber budgets? ____

____

____

____

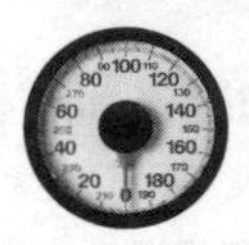

The Food-Mood Journal

If you eat to mute anger, sadness, anxiety, or stress, using this journal can weaken the powerful link between feelings and food. Why?

Once you can view emotional eating with an objective eye, you can take steps to break its hold. For example, after a few days of keeping this journal, you may notice that you eat more junk food when you're stressed or that you ate half a bag of chips when you were on the phone with your mother. With that information, you can take steps to soothe yourself with something other than food, whether it's talking with a friend or telling your mother, "I'll call you back later."

Here's how to use this journal.

At the top of the page, fill in the date and number of days you've kept your journal.

Then record everything you eat today. As you eat it, *note your mood*. Are you angry? Jealous? Agitated? Afraid? Happy? Anxious? Content? Describe that emotion in the "Mood" column. Then notice your physical position. Are you sitting on the couch watching TV? Standing next to the stove? Seated at the dining-room table? Seated at your desk at work? Record it in the "Position" column.

Last, consider the speed at which you're eating. Are you eating slowly as you enjoy the newspaper? Gulping, cramming, shoving food into your mouth? Calmly savoring each mouthful? Record it in the "How I Ate" column.

Next, check off your servings of water and fruits and vegetables. Fill in the amount of exercise you did, the number of calories you burned, and your thoughts and feelings on today's eating and exercise.

In the "Alternatives" space, brainstorm ways that you could have dealt with that emotion or other food alternatives. Could you have taken a 10-minute timeout from your tension-filled meeting so you wouldn't have grabbed that doughnut? Ducked into a bookstore during lunch instead of heading for the ice cream shop? Told the person you were angry with why you were angry?

DATE *5/5/02* **DAY** *15*

FOOD-MOOD JOURNAL
SAMPLE PAGE

Record everything you ate today:

FOOD	MOOD	POSITION	HOW I ATE
MORNING *Bagel w/cream cheese* *Coffee w/regular milk*	*Tired*	*At my desk, reading e-mail*	*Fast, without thinking*
MIDDAY *2 cups salad greens* *1 chicken breast* *1 can diet Coke*	*Happy*	*At Wendy's*	*Leisurely, with friends while chatting*
EVENING *Bowl of homemade chili w/lots of vegetables* *1 slice bread* *½ cup rice (measured)*	*Content*	*At dining-room table w/husband*	*A little fast; I always finish before he does*
SNACKS *½ carton chocolate–peanut butter ice cream*	*Upset*	*Standing in front of freezer*	*Like a possessed person—upset by argument w/ my mother*
BITES & TASTES *Several bites of chili*	*Busy*	*Making dinner*	*Right out of the pot!*

Check off each serving you had of the following:

WATER ☒ ☒ ☒ ☒ ☒ ☒ ☒ ☐

FRUITS & VEGETABLES ☒ ☒ ☒ ☐ ☐ ☐ ☐ ☐ ☐

Exercise completed today: *Rode bike for 45 min.*

Calories burned: *408*

My thoughts and feelings on today's eating and exercise: *Well, I was doing okay until the ice cream attack.*

Alternatives to what I ate today: *I need to work things out better with my mother so that we argue less.*

WEEK 1

FOOD-MOOD JOURNAL

DATE: _______ DAY: _______ WEEK-BEGINNING WEIGHT: _______

WEIGHT-LOSS TOOLS TO TRY THIS WEEK:

FOOD TOOL: Try to eat whole fruits and vegetables instead of drinking juice. They're higher in fiber, more filling, and usually contain fewer calories.

MOOD TOOL: If you tend to overeat when you're down, tell yourself that those chips and M&M's won't make you feel better. Make a list of things to do when you need a lift, such as calling a friend, taking a walk, or going to a movie. Then, when you're blue, take out your list, pick an activity, and do it.

MOVE TOOL: Add impact. While stationary bikes are good for your heart and easy on your knees, to get maximum weight-loss benefit, add some impact. To maximize your fat burn, add a day or two of jogging to your workout routine. Or simply alternate walking briskly with short bouts of jogging.

BEHAVIOR TOOL: Be a trend spotter. After 2 weeks of recording in your journal, look through it for trends and patterns. Circle supportive habits and behaviors in one color and unsupportive choices in another.

Anticipated Diet Danger Zones for this week:

____

Strategies to combat them:

____

____

Goals for the week:

____

____

Calories to burn each day with exercise: _____

MOTIVATIONAL THOUGHT FOR THE WEEK:

If you always do what you've always done, you'll always get what you always got.

—Weight Watchers International

DATE ____________ **DAY** ____________

Record everything you ate today:

FOOD	MOOD	POSITION	HOW I ATE
MORNING			
MIDDAY			
EVENING			
SNACKS			
BITES & TASTES			

Check off each serving you had of the following:

WATER ☐ ☐ ☐ ☐ ☐ ☐ ☐ ☐

FRUITS & VEGETABLES ☐ ☐ ☐ ☐ ☐ ☐ ☐ ☐ ☐

Exercise completed today: ______________________________

______________________________ **Calories burned:** __________

My thoughts and feelings on today's eating and exercise: ______________

____

Alternatives to what I ate today: ______________________________

____

DATE ______________ **DAY** 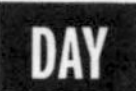

Record everything you ate today:

FOOD	MOOD	POSITION	HOW I ATE
MORNING			
MIDDAY			
EVENING			
SNACKS			
BITES & TASTES			

Check off each serving you had of the following:

WATER ☐ ☐ ☐ ☐ ☐ ☐ ☐ ☐

FRUITS & VEGETABLES ☐ ☐ ☐ ☐ ☐ ☐ ☐ ☐ ☐

Exercise completed today: ______________________________

______________________________ **Calories burned:** __________

My thoughts and feelings on today's eating and exercise: __________

____

Alternatives to what I ate today: ______________________________

____

DATE ________________ **DAY** ____________

Record everything you ate today:

FOOD	MOOD	POSITION	HOW I ATE
MORNING			
MIDDAY			
EVENING			
SNACKS			
BITES & TASTES			

Check off each serving you had of the following:

WATER ☐ ☐ ☐ ☐ ☐ ☐ ☐ ☐

FRUITS & VEGETABLES ☐ ☐ ☐ ☐ ☐ ☐ ☐ ☐ ☐

Exercise completed today: ________________________________

________________________________ **Calories burned:** __________

My thoughts and feelings on today's eating and exercise: ______________

____

Alternatives to what I ate today: ______________________________

____

DATE ____________ **DAY** ________

Record everything you ate today:

FOOD	MOOD	POSITION	HOW I ATE
MORNING			
MIDDAY			
EVENING			
SNACKS			
BITES & TASTES			

Check off each serving you had of the following:

WATER ☐ ☐ ☐ ☐ ☐ ☐ ☐ ☐

FRUITS & VEGETABLES ☐ ☐ ☐ ☐ ☐ ☐ ☐ ☐ ☐

Exercise completed today: ____________________________________

____________________________________ **Calories burned:** __________

My thoughts and feelings on today's eating and exercise: ____________

____

Alternatives to what I ate today: ______________________________

____

DATE ______________ **DAY** __________

Record everything you ate today:

FOOD	MOOD	POSITION	HOW I ATE
MORNING			
MIDDAY			
EVENING			
SNACKS			
BITES & TASTES			

Check off each serving you had of the following:

WATER ☐ ☐ ☐ ☐ ☐ ☐ ☐ ☐

FRUITS & VEGETABLES ☐ ☐ ☐ ☐ ☐ ☐ ☐ ☐ ☐

Exercise completed today: ______________________________

______________________________ **Calories burned:** __________

My thoughts and feelings on today's eating and exercise: __________

____

Alternatives to what I ate today: ______________________________

____

DATE ______________ **DAY** __________

Record everything you ate today:

FOOD	MOOD	POSITION	HOW I ATE
MORNING			
MIDDAY			
EVENING			
SNACKS			
BITES & TASTES			

Check off each serving you had of the following:

WATER ☐ ☐ ☐ ☐ ☐ ☐ ☐ ☐

FRUITS & VEGETABLES ☐ ☐ ☐ ☐ ☐ ☐ ☐ ☐ ☐

Exercise completed today: ______________________________

______________________________ **Calories burned:** __________

My thoughts and feelings on today's eating and exercise: ______________

____

Alternatives to what I ate today: ______________________________

____

DATE ______________ **DAY** __________

Record everything you ate today:

FOOD	MOOD	POSITION	HOW I ATE
MORNING			
MIDDAY			
EVENING			
SNACKS			
BITES & TASTES			

Check off each serving you had of the following:

WATER ☐ ☐ ☐ ☐ ☐ ☐ ☐ ☐

FRUITS & VEGETABLES ☐ ☐ ☐ ☐ ☐ ☐ ☐ ☐ ☐

Exercise completed today: ______________________________

______________________________ **Calories burned:** __________

My thoughts and feelings on today's eating and exercise: __________

____

Alternatives to what I ate today: ______________________________

____

Weekly Review

DATE: __________ **DAY:** _________

WEEK-ENDING WEIGHT: ______ **WEIGHT CHANGE THIS WEEK:** ______

Diet Danger Zones encountered: ________________________________

____

____

____

Most helpful tools used: ________________________________

____

____

____

Least helpful tools used: ________________________________

____

____

____

Patterns I noticed this week: ________________________________

____

____

____

This week I learned that: ________________________________

____

____

____

Trends that I noticed this week with my food and moods: ______________

____

____

____

WEEK 2

FOOD-MOOD JOURNAL

DATE: ________ DAY: ________ WEEK-BEGINNING WEIGHT: ________

WEIGHT-LOSS TOOLS TO TRY THIS WEEK:

FOOD TOOL: Go with the whole grain. Try these easy, tasty whole grain foods: quick-cooking whole grain couscous, brown rice, whole wheat pasta, wheat germ sprinkled over salad, air-popped popcorn, whole grain crackers, hot oatmeal, or grains such as millet, quinoa, and cracked wheat.

MOOD TOOL: Feeling down? Step outside. Brisk activity can relieve depression as well as the need for antidepressants. Just 30 minutes of activity three times a week is enough to bring about improvement.

MOVE TOOL: Buy two pairs of running shoes. Keep one at home and one in your office or car. You'll be ready to rack up extra miles at a moment's notice if you find some unexpected free time in your schedule.

BEHAVIOR TOOL: Add more steps to your day. Studies have shown that sedentary people who wear pedometers and have a daily goal for the number of steps they'll walk become more active all day and see improvements in fitness and body fat. Buy a pedometer—they're as low as $20—and aim to increase your number of steps to 10,000 or more.

Anticipated Diet Danger Zones for this week:

____

Strategies to combat them:

____

____

Goals for the week:

____

____

Calories to burn each day with exercise: ________

MOTIVATIONAL THOUGHT FOR THE WEEK:

There's no such thing as failure if you continue to try.
There's just unfinished business.

—Cathy Nonas, R.D.

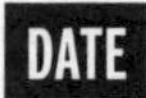

__________ **DAY** __________

Record everything you ate today:

FOOD	MOOD	POSITION	HOW I ATE
MORNING			
MIDDAY			
EVENING			
SNACKS			
BITES & TASTES			

Check off each serving you had of the following:

WATER ☐ ☐ ☐ ☐ ☐ ☐ ☐ ☐

FRUITS & VEGETABLES ☐ ☐ ☐ ☐ ☐ ☐ ☐ ☐ ☐

Exercise completed today: ______________________________

______________________________ **Calories burned:** __________

My thoughts and feelings on today's eating and exercise: __________

____

Alternatives to what I ate today: __________________________

____

DATE ____________ **DAY** ____________

Record everything you ate today:

FOOD	MOOD	POSITION	HOW I ATE
MORNING			
MIDDAY			
EVENING			
SNACKS			
BITES & TASTES			

Check off each serving you had of the following:

WATER ☐ ☐ ☐ ☐ ☐ ☐ ☐ ☐

FRUITS & VEGETABLES ☐ ☐ ☐ ☐ ☐ ☐ ☐ ☐ ☐

Exercise completed today: ______________________________

______________________________ **Calories burned:** ________

My thoughts and feelings on today's eating and exercise: ____________

____

Alternatives to what I ate today: ______________________________

____

DATE ______________ **DAY** __________

Record everything you ate today:

FOOD	MOOD	POSITION	HOW I ATE
MORNING			
MIDDAY			
EVENING			
SNACKS			
BITES & TASTES			

Check off each serving you had of the following:

WATER ☐ ☐ ☐ ☐ ☐ ☐ ☐ ☐

FRUITS & VEGETABLES ☐ ☐ ☐ ☐ ☐ ☐ ☐ ☐ ☐

Exercise completed today: ____________________________________

____________________________________ **Calories burned:** __________

My thoughts and feelings on today's eating and exercise: ______________

____

Alternatives to what I ate today: ______________________________

____

DATE ____________ **DAY** ________

Record everything you ate today:

FOOD	MOOD	POSITION	HOW I ATE
MORNING			
MIDDAY			
EVENING			
SNACKS			
BITES & TASTES			

Check off each serving you had of the following:

WATER ☐ ☐ ☐ ☐ ☐ ☐ ☐ ☐

FRUITS & VEGETABLES ☐ ☐ ☐ ☐ ☐ ☐ ☐ ☐ ☐

Exercise completed today: ____________________

____________________ **Calories burned:** ________

My thoughts and feelings on today's eating and exercise: ____________

____

Alternatives to what I ate today: ____________________

____

DATE ____________ DAY ________

Record everything you ate today:

FOOD	MOOD	POSITION	HOW I ATE
MORNING			
MIDDAY			
EVENING			
SNACKS			
BITES & TASTES			

Check off each serving you had of the following:

WATER ☐ ☐ ☐ ☐ ☐ ☐ ☐ ☐

FRUITS & VEGETABLES ☐ ☐ ☐ ☐ ☐ ☐ ☐ ☐ ☐

Exercise completed today: ____________________________________

____________________________________ **Calories burned:** __________

My thoughts and feelings on today's eating and exercise: __________

____

Alternatives to what I ate today: ______________________________

____

DATE ______________ **DAY** __________

Record everything you ate today:

FOOD	MOOD	POSITION	HOW I ATE
MORNING			
MIDDAY			
EVENING			
SNACKS			
BITES & TASTES			

Check off each serving you had of the following:

WATER ☐ ☐ ☐ ☐ ☐ ☐ ☐ ☐

FRUITS & VEGETABLES ☐ ☐ ☐ ☐ ☐ ☐ ☐ ☐ ☐

Exercise completed today: ______________________________________

______________________________________ **Calories burned:** __________

My thoughts and feelings on today's eating and exercise: ______________

____

Alternatives to what I ate today: ______________________________

____

DATE ____________ **DAY** ________

Record everything you ate today:

FOOD	MOOD	POSITION	HOW I ATE
MORNING			
MIDDAY			
EVENING			
SNACKS			
BITES & TASTES			

Check off each serving you had of the following:

WATER ☐ ☐ ☐ ☐ ☐ ☐ ☐ ☐

FRUITS & VEGETABLES ☐ ☐ ☐ ☐ ☐ ☐ ☐ ☐ ☐

Exercise completed today: ______________________________

______________________________ **Calories burned:** ________

My thoughts and feelings on today's eating and exercise: ____________

____

Alternatives to what I ate today: ______________________

____

Weekly Review

DATE: ________ **DAY:** ________

WEEK-ENDING WEIGHT: ______ **WEIGHT CHANGE THIS WEEK:** ______

Diet Danger Zones encountered: ______________________________

____

____

____

Most helpful tools used: ______________________________

____

____

____

Least helpful tools used: ______________________________

____

____

____

Patterns I noticed this week: ______________________________

____

____

____

This week I learned that: ______________________________

____

____

____

Trends that I noticed this week with my food and moods: ______________

____

____

____

WEEK 3

FOOD-MOOD JOURNAL

DATE: ______ DAY: ______ WEEK-BEGINNING WEIGHT: ______

WEIGHT-LOSS TOOLS TO TRY THIS WEEK:

FOOD TOOL: Rather than food, focus on fun! For example, if you're at a picnic, play Frisbee to keep yourself from eating a hamburger—you'll save 528 calories. If you don't buy popcorn before the movie starts, you may be more likely to buy the smaller size if you get up in the middle of the movie—or you may end up not buying it at all, a savings of 264 to 900 calories.

MOOD TOOL: Stress less. Learn a stress-reducing technique, such as meditation or deep breathing, and be sure you get enough sleep.

MOVE TOOL: Set an exercise goal instead of a weight-loss goal, such as walking your first 5-K, hiking to the nearest mountain summit, or beating your husband in tennis. Striving toward that goal will help you lose weight as well.

BEHAVIOR TOOL: Lose your membership in the clean-plate club. If you don't want to finish the food on your plate, throw it away. Although our parents made us feel guilty about the starving children in other parts of the world, you know now that finishing a second helping of tuna noodle casserole isn't going to help them.

Anticipated Diet Danger Zones for this week:

____

Strategies to combat them:

____

____

Goals for the week:

____

____

Calories to burn each day with exercise: ______

MOTIVATIONAL THOUGHT FOR THE WEEK:

Love your body as it is. It's tough to take care of something that you hate!

—Cyberdiet.com

DATE ____________ **DAY** ____________

Record everything you ate today:

FOOD	MOOD	POSITION	HOW I ATE
MORNING			
MIDDAY			
EVENING			
SNACKS			
BITES & TASTES			

Check off each serving you had of the following:

WATER ☐ ☐ ☐ ☐ ☐ ☐ ☐ ☐

FRUITS & VEGETABLES ☐ ☐ ☐ ☐ ☐ ☐ ☐ ☐ ☐

Exercise completed today: ____________________

____________________ **Calories burned:** __________

My thoughts and feelings on today's eating and exercise: ____________________

____

Alternatives to what I ate today: ____________________

____

DATE ____________ **DAY** ________

Record everything you ate today:

FOOD	MOOD	POSITION	HOW I ATE
MORNING			
MIDDAY			
EVENING			
SNACKS			
BITES & TASTES			

Check off each serving you had of the following:

WATER ☐ ☐ ☐ ☐ ☐ ☐ ☐ ☐

FRUITS & VEGETABLES ☐ ☐ ☐ ☐ ☐ ☐ ☐ ☐ ☐

Exercise completed today: ______________________________

______________________________ **Calories burned:** ________

My thoughts and feelings on today's eating and exercise: ____________

____

Alternatives to what I ate today: ______________________________

____

DATE ____________ **DAY** ________

Record everything you ate today:

FOOD	MOOD	POSITION	HOW I ATE
MORNING			
MIDDAY			
EVENING			
SNACKS			
BITES & TASTES			

Check off each serving you had of the following:

WATER ☐ ☐ ☐ ☐ ☐ ☐ ☐ ☐

FRUITS & VEGETABLES ☐ ☐ ☐ ☐ ☐ ☐ ☐ ☐ ☐

Exercise completed today: ______________________________

______________________________ **Calories burned:** ________

My thoughts and feelings on today's eating and exercise: ________

____

Alternatives to what I ate today: ______________________________

____

DATE ____________ **DAY** ________

Record everything you ate today:

FOOD	MOOD	POSITION	HOW I ATE
MORNING			
MIDDAY			
EVENING			
SNACKS			
BITES & TASTES			

Check off each serving you had of the following:

WATER ☐ ☐ ☐ ☐ ☐ ☐ ☐ ☐

FRUITS & VEGETABLES ☐ ☐ ☐ ☐ ☐ ☐ ☐ ☐ ☐

Exercise completed today: ____________________________

____________________________ **Calories burned:** ________

My thoughts and feelings on today's eating and exercise: ____________

____

Alternatives to what I ate today: ____________________________

____

DATE ____________ **DAY** ________

Record everything you ate today:

FOOD	MOOD	POSITION	HOW I ATE
MORNING			
MIDDAY			
EVENING			
SNACKS			
BITES & TASTES			

Check off each serving you had of the following:

WATER ☐ ☐ ☐ ☐ ☐ ☐ ☐ ☐

FRUITS & VEGETABLES ☐ ☐ ☐ ☐ ☐ ☐ ☐ ☐ ☐

Exercise completed today: ____________________________

____________________________ **Calories burned:** ________

My thoughts and feelings on today's eating and exercise: ____________

____

Alternatives to what I ate today: ____________________________

____

DATE ______________ **DAY** __________

Record everything you ate today:

FOOD	MOOD	POSITION	HOW I ATE
MORNING			
MIDDAY			
EVENING			
SNACKS			
BITES & TASTES			

Check off each serving you had of the following:

WATER ☐ ☐ ☐ ☐ ☐ ☐ ☐ ☐

FRUITS & VEGETABLES ☐ ☐ ☐ ☐ ☐ ☐ ☐ ☐ ☐

Exercise completed today: ____________________________________

____________________________________ **Calories burned:** __________

My thoughts and feelings on today's eating and exercise: __________

____

Alternatives to what I ate today: ______________________________

____

DATE ____________ **DAY** ________

Record everything you ate today:

FOOD	MOOD	POSITION	HOW I ATE
MORNING			
MIDDAY			
EVENING			
SNACKS			
BITES & TASTES			

Check off each serving you had of the following:

WATER ☐ ☐ ☐ ☐ ☐ ☐ ☐ ☐

FRUITS & VEGETABLES ☐ ☐ ☐ ☐ ☐ ☐ ☐ ☐ ☐

Exercise completed today: ______________________________

______________________________ **Calories burned:** ________

My thoughts and feelings on today's eating and exercise: ____________

____

Alternatives to what I ate today: ______________________________

____

Weekly Review

DATE: __________ DAY: _________

WEEK-ENDING WEIGHT: ______ WEIGHT CHANGE THIS WEEK: ______

Diet Danger Zones encountered: ____

____

____

____

Most helpful tools used: ____

____

____

____

Least helpful tools used: ____

____

____

____

Patterns I noticed this week: ____

____

____

____

This week I learned that: ____

____

____

____

Trends that I noticed this week with my food and moods: ______________

____

____

____

WEEK 4

FOOD-MOOD JOURNAL

DATE: _______ DAY: _______ WEEK-BEGINNING WEIGHT: _______

WEIGHT-LOSS TOOLS TO TRY THIS WEEK:

FOOD TOOL: Increase your fiber intake. To get more of the rough stuff, make these simple switches: 1 cup of raisin bran (8 g) instead of 1 cup of Cocoa Puffs (0 g); ½ cup of baked beans (7 g) instead of ½ cup of pasta salad (1 g); 1 large apple (7 g) instead of a fruit rollup (0 g); 1 cup of lentil soup (7 g) instead of 1 cup of chicken with rice soup (1 g).

MOOD TOOL: Do you find yourself down in the dumps, which makes you eat more? Try this strategy to feel better about your life. Start a gratitude journal. In another notebook or even within the pages of this diary, each day write down something you're grateful for: a sunny day, a lunch date with a friend, the way your cat purrs when she twines around your ankles.

MOVE TOOL: Are your feet sore from walking, jogging, or other workout-related aches and pains? Treat yourself to an at-home pedicure.

BEHAVIOR TOOL: If you look in the mirror and see nothing but your flaws, start naming one positive trait that you have for each negative one.

Anticipated Diet Danger Zones for this week:

____

Strategies to combat them:

____

____

Goals for the week:

____

____

Calories to burn each day with exercise: _______

MOTIVATIONAL THOUGHT FOR THE WEEK:

Don't give up what you want the most for what you want at the moment!

—Weight Watchers International

DATE ____________ **DAY** ________

Record everything you ate today:

FOOD	MOOD	POSITION	HOW I ATE
MORNING			
MIDDAY			
EVENING			
SNACKS			
BITES & TASTES			

Check off each serving you had of the following:

WATER ☐ ☐ ☐ ☐ ☐ ☐ ☐ ☐

FRUITS & VEGETABLES ☐ ☐ ☐ ☐ ☐ ☐ ☐ ☐ ☐

Exercise completed today: ______________________________

______________________________ **Calories burned:** ________

My thoughts and feelings on today's eating and exercise: ____________

____

Alternatives to what I ate today: ______________________________

____

DATE ____________ DAY ________

Record everything you ate today:

FOOD	MOOD	POSITION	HOW I ATE
MORNING			
MIDDAY			
EVENING			
SNACKS			
BITES & TASTES			

Check off each serving you had of the following:

WATER ☐ ☐ ☐ ☐ ☐ ☐ ☐ ☐

FRUITS & VEGETABLES ☐ ☐ ☐ ☐ ☐ ☐ ☐ ☐ ☐

Exercise completed today: ______________________________

______________________________ **Calories burned:** ________

My thoughts and feelings on today's eating and exercise: ________

____

Alternatives to what I ate today: ______________________________

____

DATE ______________ DAY __________

Record everything you ate today:

FOOD	MOOD	POSITION	HOW I ATE
MORNING			
MIDDAY			
EVENING			
SNACKS			
BITES & TASTES			

Check off each serving you had of the following:

WATER ☐ ☐ ☐ ☐ ☐ ☐ ☐ ☐

FRUITS & VEGETABLES ☐ ☐ ☐ ☐ ☐ ☐ ☐ ☐ ☐

Exercise completed today: ____

____ **Calories burned:** __________

My thoughts and feelings on today's eating and exercise: ______________

____

Alternatives to what I ate today: __________________________________

____

DATE ____________ **DAY** ________

Record everything you ate today:

FOOD	MOOD	POSITION	HOW I ATE
MORNING			
MIDDAY			
EVENING			
SNACKS			
BITES & TASTES			

Check off each serving you had of the following:

WATER ☐ ☐ ☐ ☐ ☐ ☐ ☐ ☐

FRUITS & VEGETABLES ☐ ☐ ☐ ☐ ☐ ☐ ☐ ☐ ☐

Exercise completed today: ________________________________

________________________________ **Calories burned:** ________

My thoughts and feelings on today's eating and exercise: ________

____

Alternatives to what I ate today: ________________________

____

DATE ______________ **DAY** ________

Record everything you ate today:

FOOD	MOOD	POSITION	HOW I ATE
MORNING			
MIDDAY			
EVENING			
SNACKS			
BITES & TASTES			

Check off each serving you had of the following:

WATER ☐ ☐ ☐ ☐ ☐ ☐ ☐ ☐

FRUITS & VEGETABLES ☐ ☐ ☐ ☐ ☐ ☐ ☐ ☐ ☐

Exercise completed today: ______________________________

______________________________ **Calories burned:** ________

My thoughts and feelings on today's eating and exercise: ____________

____

Alternatives to what I ate today: ______________________________

____

DATE ____________ **DAY** ________

Record everything you ate today:

FOOD	MOOD	POSITION	HOW I ATE
MORNING			
MIDDAY			
EVENING			
SNACKS			
BITES & TASTES			

Check off each serving you had of the following:

WATER ☐ ☐ ☐ ☐ ☐ ☐ ☐ ☐

FRUITS & VEGETABLES ☐ ☐ ☐ ☐ ☐ ☐ ☐ ☐ ☐

Exercise completed today: ________________________________

________________________________ **Calories burned:** __________

My thoughts and feelings on today's eating and exercise: ____________

____

Alternatives to what I ate today: ________________________________

____

DATE ________________ **DAY** __________

Record everything you ate today:

FOOD	MOOD	POSITION	HOW I ATE
MORNING			
MIDDAY			
EVENING			
SNACKS			
BITES & TASTES			

Check off each serving you had of the following:

WATER ☐ ☐ ☐ ☐ ☐ ☐ ☐ ☐

FRUITS & VEGETABLES ☐ ☐ ☐ ☐ ☐ ☐ ☐ ☐ ☐

Exercise completed today: ________________________________

________________________________ **Calories burned:** __________

My thoughts and feelings on today's eating and exercise: __________

____

Alternatives to what I ate today: ________________________

____

Weekly Review

DATE: __________ DAY: _________

WEEK-ENDING WEIGHT: ______ WEIGHT CHANGE THIS WEEK: ______

Diet Danger Zones encountered: ________________________________

____

____

____

Most helpful tools used: ________________________________

____

____

____

Least helpful tools used: ________________________________

____

____

____

Patterns I noticed this week: ________________________________

____

____

____

This week I learned that: ________________________________

____

____

____

Trends that I noticed this week with my food and moods: ______________

____

____

____

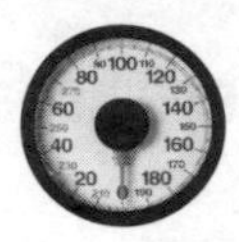

The Portion-Control Journal

This is what the experts say you should eat each day: six to eight servings of grains; at least five servings of fruits and vegetables; two to three servings of high-calcium foods; two to four servings of lean meat, fish, poultry, and eggs; one to two servings of legumes, nuts, or seeds; and 2 tablespoons of monounsaturated fat such as olive or canola oil.

How do you do all this? How do you get it right? What exactly is a serving size? And is there room for any good stuff?

The Portion-Control Journal puts everything into perspective. The portions are divided into categories of food. But unlike Weight Watchers or the exchanges that you are used to (or the Food Guide Pyramid, for that matter), here they're broken up into seven categories: grains (starches); fruits and vegetables; high-calcium foods; lean meats, poultry, and eggs; fish; legumes, nuts, and seeds; and fat. You will see that some of the foods (such as sardines) are in both the fish and high-calcium categories. You will also see that high-fat meats, cheeses, and saturated oils, as well as what you could call "junk" or uncountable foods, are missing. Therefore, if you follow these categories, you will have a nutrient-rich but low-calorie day.

The list below is an incomplete (but adequate) idea of what to do and how to proceed. Total calories are between 1,300 and 1,600.

If you have calorie room left for any other food that does not fit into these categories, like a candy bar, or foods that defy characterization, like wonton soup, record it on the "I dunno" line.

Below you'll find the standard low-calorie serving sizes of each category. An asterisk indicates that the food is higher in fat and therefore higher in calories.

GRAINS (STARCHES):

Choose six to eight (all except the bagel are high in fiber).

1 slice any bread with 2 or more grams of fiber
1 ounce cereal with more than 3 grams of fiber

¼ bagel
⅓ cup brown rice, quinoa, or millet
½ cup soba noodles
1 medium sweet or regular potato
1 ear corn

FRUITS AND VEGETABLES:

Choose at least five (foods in this category, particularly vegetables, are excellent fillers if you are hungry or a volume eater).

1 cup any raw vegetables
½ cup any cooked vegetable
1 cup berries
1 small apple or orange
½ grapefruit or banana
15 grapes
½ cantaloupe
¼ cup dried fruit

HIGH-CALCIUM FOODS:

Choose two to three (each serving supplies about 300 milligrams of calcium).

1 cup fat-free milk (or any other kind*)
1 cup plain fat-free yogurt
1 cup fat-free soy milk (calcium-fortified)
1½ ounces cheese*
8 ounces tofu
3 ounces sardines with bones
1 cup collard greens
½ cup ricotta cheese

LEAN MEATS, POULTRY, AND EGGS:

Choose one or two.

3 ounces cooked lean meat or skinless poultry
2 eggs

FISH:

Choose one or two.

3–4 ounces any fish other than shellfish
6 ounces shellfish

LEGUMES, NUTS, AND SEEDS:

Choose one or two.

½ cup cooked beans
2 tablespoons nuts*

FAT:

Choose two.

1 tablespoon olive oil
1 tablespoon canola oil

In addition to checking off the boxes, fill out the remaining portions of the journal: the exercise you completed today, the number of calories you burned, and your thoughts and feeling on today's eating and exercise.

DATE *6/5/02*

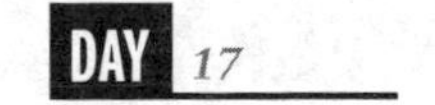

PORTION-CONTROL JOURNAL

SAMPLE PAGE

CHECK OFF EACH SERVING YOU EAT OF THE FOLLOWING:
GRAINS (STARCHES) [X] [X] [X] [X] [X] [X] [ ] [ ]
FRUITS AND VEGETABLES [X] [X] [X] [X] [X]
HIGH-CALCIUM FOODS [X] [ ] [ ]
LEAN MEATS, POULTRY, AND EGGS [X] [X]
FISH [X] [ ]
LEGUMES, NUTS, AND SEEDS [X] [ ]
FAT [X] [X]
WATER [X] [X] [X] [X] [X] [X] [X] [ ]

Record any foods that don't fit into the above categories and any "I dunno" foods:

FOOD	CALORIES
10 pretzels	*229*
2 Tbsp. butter	*202*
2 bites leftover Chinese food	*28*
	Total: *459*

What percentage of your food today was "I dunno" foods? *Around 5%*

Exercise completed today: *Walked to the grocery store and back for 1 hour. Cleaned house for 1 hour.* **Calories burned:** *204*

My thoughts and feelings on today's eating and exercise: *I checked off a lot of boxes today, and almost everything I ate fit into the portion categories. I'm also pleased that I walked for an hour and cleaned my house to boot!*

WEEK 1

PORTION-CONTROL JOURNAL

DATE: ________ DAY: _______ WEEK-BEGINNING WEIGHT: ________

WEIGHT-LOSS TOOLS TO TRY THIS WEEK:

FOOD TOOL: The following items are great for adding flavor, moisture, texture, and versatility to every meal, and they're low in calories: Dijon and Pommery mustards, balsamic and wine vinegars, sauces like salsa, tamari, and soy, and herbs and spices.

MOOD TOOL: Need more motivation? Think of all the reasons why you want to be your healthiest self. Maybe you want to go off your blood-pressure medication. Maybe you want to live to see your grandchildren grow up.

MOVE TOOL: Exercising but not seeing the improvements you want? Try a fitness trainer. Rates can be as low as $20 per hour, and even a few sessions can make a difference. To find certified trainers in your area, contact the American Council on Exercise at (800) 825-3636 or the National Strength and Conditioning Association at (800) 815-6826.

BEHAVIOR TOOL: Is your schedule so busy you succumb to fast-food temptations on the way home from work? Take a look at your days and design some formulaic meals: a turkey sandwich at lunch, a frozen low-calorie meal at dinner, a Slim-Fast drink in the afternoon. The planning is the most difficult. So get that part over with and go with the flow.

Anticipated Diet Danger Zones for this week:

____

Strategies to combat them:

____

____

Goals for the week:

____

____

Calories to burn each day with exercise: ________

MOTIVATIONAL THOUGHT FOR THE WEEK:

Not losing weight but not gaining either?
Celebrate, for that too is a victory!

—Cyberdiet.com

DATE ____________ **DAY** ____________

CHECK OFF EACH SERVING YOU EAT OF THE FOLLOWING:
GRAINS (STARCHES) ☐ ☐ ☐ ☐ ☐ ☐ ☐ ☐
FRUITS AND VEGETABLES ☐ ☐ ☐ ☐ ☐
HIGH-CALCIUM FOODS ☐ ☐ ☐
LEAN MEATS, POULTRY, AND EGGS ☐ ☐
FISH ☐ ☐
LEGUMES, NUTS, AND SEEDS ☐ ☐
FAT ☐ ☐
WATER ☐ ☐ ☐ ☐ ☐ ☐ ☐ ☐

Record any foods that don't fit into the above categories and any "I dunno" foods:

FOOD	CALORIES
	Total:

What percentage of your food today was "I dunno" foods? ____________

Exercise completed today: ____________________________________

____________________________________ **Calories burned:** ____________

My thoughts and feelings on today's eating and exercise: ____________

____

____

____

DATE ______________ **DAY** ______________

CHECK OFF EACH SERVING YOU EAT OF THE FOLLOWING:
GRAINS (STARCHES) ☐ ☐ ☐ ☐ ☐ ☐ ☐ ☐
FRUITS AND VEGETABLES ☐ ☐ ☐ ☐ ☐
HIGH-CALCIUM FOODS ☐ ☐ ☐
LEAN MEATS, POULTRY, AND EGGS ☐ ☐
FISH ☐ ☐
LEGUMES, NUTS, AND SEEDS ☐ ☐
FAT ☐ ☐
WATER ☐ ☐ ☐ ☐ ☐ ☐ ☐ ☐

Record any foods that don't fit into the above categories and any "I dunno" foods:

FOOD	CALORIES
	Total:

What percentage of your food today was "I dunno" foods? ______________

Exercise completed today: ____

____ **Calories burned:** __________

My thoughts and feelings on today's eating and exercise: ______________

____

____

____

DATE ____________ **DAY** ____________

CHECK OFF EACH SERVING YOU EAT OF THE FOLLOWING:
GRAINS (STARCHES) ☐ ☐ ☐ ☐ ☐ ☐ ☐ ☐
FRUITS AND VEGETABLES ☐ ☐ ☐ ☐ ☐
HIGH-CALCIUM FOODS ☐ ☐ ☐
LEAN MEATS, POULTRY, AND EGGS ☐ ☐
FISH ☐ ☐
LEGUMES, NUTS, AND SEEDS ☐ ☐
FAT ☐ ☐
WATER ☐ ☐ ☐ ☐ ☐ ☐ ☐ ☐

Record any foods that don't fit into the above categories and any "I dunno" foods:

FOOD	CALORIES
	Total:

What percentage of your food today was "I dunno" foods? ____________

Exercise completed today: ____

____ **Calories burned:** ____________

My thoughts and feelings on today's eating and exercise: ____________

____

____

____

DATE ____________ **DAY** ____________

CHECK OFF EACH SERVING YOU EAT OF THE FOLLOWING:
GRAINS (STARCHES) ☐ ☐ ☐ ☐ ☐ ☐ ☐ ☐
FRUITS AND VEGETABLES ☐ ☐ ☐ ☐ ☐
HIGH-CALCIUM FOODS ☐ ☐ ☐
LEAN MEATS, POULTRY, AND EGGS ☐ ☐
FISH ☐ ☐
LEGUMES, NUTS, AND SEEDS ☐ ☐
FAT ☐ ☐
WATER ☐ ☐ ☐ ☐ ☐ ☐ ☐ ☐

Record any foods that don't fit into the above categories and any "I dunno" foods:

FOOD	CALORIES
	Total:

What percentage of your food today was "I dunno" foods? ____________

Exercise completed today: ____

____ **Calories burned:** ____________

My thoughts and feelings on today's eating and exercise: ____________

____

____

____

DATE ____________ **DAY** ____________

CHECK OFF EACH SERVING YOU EAT OF THE FOLLOWING:
GRAINS (STARCHES) ☐ ☐ ☐ ☐ ☐ ☐ ☐ ☐
FRUITS AND VEGETABLES ☐ ☐ ☐ ☐ ☐
HIGH-CALCIUM FOODS ☐ ☐ ☐
LEAN MEATS, POULTRY, AND EGGS ☐ ☐
FISH ☐ ☐
LEGUMES, NUTS, AND SEEDS ☐ ☐
FAT ☐ ☐
WATER ☐ ☐ ☐ ☐ ☐ ☐ ☐ ☐

Record any foods that don't fit into the above categories and any "I dunno" foods:

FOOD	CALORIES
	Total:

What percentage of your food today was "I dunno" foods? ____________

Exercise completed today: ________________________________

________________________________ **Calories burned:** ____________

My thoughts and feelings on today's eating and exercise: ____________

____

____

____

DATE ____________ **DAY** ____________

CHECK OFF EACH SERVING YOU EAT OF THE FOLLOWING:
GRAINS (STARCHES) ☐ ☐ ☐ ☐ ☐ ☐ ☐ ☐
FRUITS AND VEGETABLES ☐ ☐ ☐ ☐ ☐
HIGH-CALCIUM FOODS ☐ ☐ ☐
LEAN MEATS, POULTRY, AND EGGS ☐ ☐
FISH ☐ ☐
LEGUMES, NUTS, AND SEEDS ☐ ☐
FAT ☐ ☐
WATER ☐ ☐ ☐ ☐ ☐ ☐ ☐ ☐

Record any foods that don't fit into the above categories and any "I dunno" foods:

FOOD	CALORIES
	Total:

What percentage of your food today was "I dunno" foods? ____________

Exercise completed today: ______________________________

______________________________ **Calories burned:** ____________

My thoughts and feelings on today's eating and exercise: ____________

____

____

____

DATE ______________ **DAY** ______________

CHECK OFF EACH SERVING YOU EAT OF THE FOLLOWING:
GRAINS (STARCHES) ☐ ☐ ☐ ☐ ☐ ☐ ☐ ☐
FRUITS AND VEGETABLES ☐ ☐ ☐ ☐ ☐
HIGH-CALCIUM FOODS ☐ ☐ ☐
LEAN MEATS, POULTRY, AND EGGS ☐ ☐
FISH ☐ ☐
LEGUMES, NUTS, AND SEEDS ☐ ☐
FAT ☐ ☐
WATER ☐ ☐ ☐ ☐ ☐ ☐ ☐ ☐

Record any foods that don't fit into the above categories and any "I dunno" foods:

FOOD	CALORIES
	Total:

What percentage of your food today was "I dunno" foods? ______________

Exercise completed today: ____

____ **Calories burned:** __________

My thoughts and feelings on today's eating and exercise: ______________

____

____

____

Weekly Review

DATE: __________ DAY: _________

WEEK-ENDING WEIGHT: ______ WEIGHT CHANGE THIS WEEK: ______

Diet Danger Zones encountered:

Most helpful tools used:

Least helpful tools used:

Patterns I noticed this week:

This week I learned that:

Trends that I noticed this week with my portion control and extra "I dunno" foods:

WEEK 2

PORTION-CONTROL JOURNAL

DATE: _______ DAY: _______ WEEK-BEGINNING WEIGHT: _______

WEIGHT-LOSS TOOLS TO TRY THIS WEEK:

FOOD TOOL: Drink as much water as you can. Besides aiding weight loss, water reduces the risk of kidney stones, constipation, and dehydration. Drink 8 to 12 glasses of fluid each day; 5 or more should be water.

MOOD TOOL: Cheer yourself along by giving yourself a catchy nickname or adopting a motto. One woman thinks of herself as "Slim-Fast" because her friends say each time they see her, she looks thinner. Another uses the motto: "I deserve to eat healthy foods."

MOVE TOOL: Obstacle: no time. The new physical activity guidelines are different. They suggest that you start slowly and that you accumulate 30 minutes of activity each day. That means you can do 10 minutes three times each day. There's always time when you look at it from that perspective.

BEHAVIOR TOOL: Sit back in your chair when you have food in front of you. It will slow down your eating because you will have to purposefully move forward before you can eat.

Anticipated Diet Danger Zones for this week:

____

Strategies to combat them:

____

____

Goals for the week:

____

____

Calories to burn each day with exercise: _______

MOTIVATIONAL THOUGHT FOR THE WEEK:

Eat less, move more, and drown yourself in water.

—Cyberdiet.com

DATE ______ 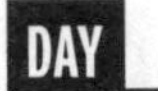 ______

CHECK OFF EACH SERVING YOU EAT OF THE FOLLOWING:
GRAINS (STARCHES) ☐ ☐ ☐ ☐ ☐ ☐ ☐ ☐
FRUITS AND VEGETABLES ☐ ☐ ☐ ☐ ☐
HIGH-CALCIUM FOODS ☐ ☐ ☐
LEAN MEATS, POULTRY, AND EGGS ☐ ☐
FISH ☐ ☐
LEGUMES, NUTS, AND SEEDS ☐ ☐
FAT ☐ ☐
WATER ☐ ☐ ☐ ☐ ☐ ☐ ☐ ☐

Record any foods that don't fit into the above categories and any "I dunno" foods:

FOOD	CALORIES
	Total:

What percentage of your food today was "I dunno" foods? ______

Exercise completed today: ______

______ **Calories burned:** ______

My thoughts and feelings on today's eating and exercise: ______

______

______

______

DATE ____________ DAY ____________

CHECK OFF EACH SERVING YOU EAT OF THE FOLLOWING:
GRAINS (STARCHES) ☐ ☐ ☐ ☐ ☐ ☐ ☐ ☐
FRUITS AND VEGETABLES ☐ ☐ ☐ ☐ ☐
HIGH-CALCIUM FOODS ☐ ☐ ☐
LEAN MEATS, POULTRY, AND EGGS ☐ ☐
FISH ☐ ☐
LEGUMES, NUTS, AND SEEDS ☐ ☐
FAT ☐ ☐
WATER ☐ ☐ ☐ ☐ ☐ ☐ ☐ ☐

Record any foods that don't fit into the above categories and any "I dunno" foods:

FOOD	CALORIES
	Total:

What percentage of your food today was "I dunno" foods? ____________

Exercise completed today: ____________________________________

____________________________________ **Calories burned:** ____________

My thoughts and feelings on today's eating and exercise: ____________

____

____

____

DATE ____________ DAY ____________

CHECK OFF EACH SERVING YOU EAT OF THE FOLLOWING:
GRAINS (STARCHES) ☐ ☐ ☐ ☐ ☐ ☐ ☐ ☐
FRUITS AND VEGETABLES ☐ ☐ ☐ ☐ ☐
HIGH-CALCIUM FOODS ☐ ☐ ☐
LEAN MEATS, POULTRY, AND EGGS ☐ ☐
FISH ☐ ☐
LEGUMES, NUTS, AND SEEDS ☐ ☐
FAT ☐ ☐
WATER ☐ ☐ ☐ ☐ ☐ ☐ ☐ ☐

Record any foods that don't fit into the above categories and any "I dunno" foods:

FOOD	CALORIES
	Total:

What percentage of your food today was "I dunno" foods? ____________

Exercise completed today: ____________

____________ **Calories burned:** ____________

My thoughts and feelings on today's eating and exercise: ____________

____

____

____

DATE ____________ DAY ____________

CHECK OFF EACH SERVING YOU EAT OF THE FOLLOWING:
GRAINS (STARCHES) ☐ ☐ ☐ ☐ ☐ ☐ ☐ ☐
FRUITS AND VEGETABLES ☐ ☐ ☐ ☐ ☐
HIGH-CALCIUM FOODS ☐ ☐ ☐
LEAN MEATS, POULTRY, AND EGGS ☐ ☐
FISH ☐ ☐
LEGUMES, NUTS, AND SEEDS ☐ ☐
FAT ☐ ☐
WATER ☐ ☐ ☐ ☐ ☐ ☐ ☐ ☐

Record any foods that don't fit into the above categories and any "I dunno" foods:

FOOD	CALORIES
	Total:

What percentage of your food today was "I dunno" foods?____________

Exercise completed today: ______________________________

______________________________ Calories burned: __________

My thoughts and feelings on today's eating and exercise: ____________

____

____

____

DATE ____________ **DAY** __________

CHECK OFF EACH SERVING YOU EAT OF THE FOLLOWING:
GRAINS (STARCHES) ☐ ☐ ☐ ☐ ☐ ☐ ☐ ☐
FRUITS AND VEGETABLES ☐ ☐ ☐ ☐ ☐
HIGH-CALCIUM FOODS ☐ ☐ ☐
LEAN MEATS, POULTRY, AND EGGS ☐ ☐
FISH ☐ ☐
LEGUMES, NUTS, AND SEEDS ☐ ☐
FAT ☐ ☐
WATER ☐ ☐ ☐ ☐ ☐ ☐ ☐ ☐

Record any foods that don't fit into the above categories and any "I dunno" foods:

FOOD	CALORIES
	Total:

What percentage of your food today was "I dunno" foods?____________

Exercise completed today: ______________________________________

______________________________________ **Calories burned:** __________

My thoughts and feelings on today's eating and exercise: ____________

____

____

____

DATE ____________ **DAY** ____________

CHECK OFF EACH SERVING YOU EAT OF THE FOLLOWING:
GRAINS (STARCHES) ☐ ☐ ☐ ☐ ☐ ☐ ☐ ☐
FRUITS AND VEGETABLES ☐ ☐ ☐ ☐ ☐
HIGH-CALCIUM FOODS ☐ ☐ ☐
LEAN MEATS, POULTRY, AND EGGS ☐ ☐
FISH ☐ ☐
LEGUMES, NUTS, AND SEEDS ☐ ☐
FAT ☐ ☐
WATER ☐ ☐ ☐ ☐ ☐ ☐ ☐ ☐

Record any foods that don't fit into the above categories and any "I dunno" foods:

FOOD	CALORIES
	Total:

What percentage of your food today was "I dunno" foods? ____________

Exercise completed today: ____________________________

____________________________ **Calories burned:** ____________

My thoughts and feelings on today's eating and exercise: ____________

____

____

____

DATE ____________ **DAY** ____________

CHECK OFF EACH SERVING YOU EAT OF THE FOLLOWING:
GRAINS (STARCHES) ☐ ☐ ☐ ☐ ☐ ☐ ☐ ☐
FRUITS AND VEGETABLES ☐ ☐ ☐ ☐ ☐
HIGH-CALCIUM FOODS ☐ ☐ ☐
LEAN MEATS, POULTRY, AND EGGS ☐ ☐
FISH ☐ ☐
LEGUMES, NUTS, AND SEEDS ☐ ☐
FAT ☐ ☐
WATER ☐ ☐ ☐ ☐ ☐ ☐ ☐ ☐

Record any foods that don't fit into the above categories and any "I dunno" foods:

FOOD	CALORIES
	Total:

What percentage of your food today was "I dunno" foods? ____________

Exercise completed today: ________________________________

________________________________ **Calories burned:** ____________

My thoughts and feelings on today's eating and exercise: ____________

____

____

____

Weekly Review

DATE: _________ DAY: ________

WEEK-ENDING WEIGHT: ______ WEIGHT CHANGE THIS WEEK: ______

Diet Danger Zones encountered: ______________________________

____

____

____

Most helpful tools used: ______________________________

____

____

____

Least helpful tools used: ______________________________

____

____

____

Patterns I noticed this week: ______________________________

____

____

____

This week I learned that: ______________________________

____

____

____

Trends that I noticed this week with my portion control and extra "I dunno" foods: ______________________________

____

____

____

WEEK 3

PORTION-CONTROL JOURNAL

DATE: ________ **DAY:** ________ **WEEK-BEGINNING WEIGHT:** ________

WEIGHT-LOSS TOOLS TO TRY THIS WEEK:

FOOD TOOL: Eat spicy foods. A few studies from Japan have shown that eating a fiery red pepper–spiced meal may boost your metabolism up to 30 percent (and reduce your desire to eat more). One caveat, they used a lot of red pepper—between 5 and 6 teaspoons per meal.

MOOD TOOL: Try wearing a bright scarf or colorful pin to help display your sunny disposition.

MOVE TOOL: Try mall walking! Some malls have formalized programs that you join to track your progress, meet other mall walkers, and even receive coupons and discounts from mall merchants. If your local mall doesn't have one, start your own club!

BEHAVIOR TOOL: Get others hooked on your healthy habits. Not only will you have the tremendous satisfaction of knowing you're helping a loved one be healthier, but you'll also gain a new supporter.

Anticipated Diet Danger Zones for this week:

____

Strategies to combat them:

____

____

Goals for the week:

____

____

Calories to burn each day with exercise: ________

MOTIVATIONAL THOUGHT FOR THE WEEK:

There is no Skinny Fairy; there's no magic to weight loss.

DATE ____________ **DAY** ________

CHECK OFF EACH SERVING YOU EAT OF THE FOLLOWING:
GRAINS (STARCHES) ☐ ☐ ☐ ☐ ☐ ☐ ☐ ☐
FRUITS AND VEGETABLES ☐ ☐ ☐ ☐ ☐
HIGH-CALCIUM FOODS ☐ ☐ ☐
LEAN MEATS, POULTRY, AND EGGS ☐ ☐
FISH ☐ ☐
LEGUMES, NUTS, AND SEEDS ☐ ☐
FAT ☐ ☐
WATER ☐ ☐ ☐ ☐ ☐ ☐ ☐ ☐

Record any foods that don't fit into the above categories and any "I dunno" foods:

FOOD	CALORIES
	Total:

What percentage of your food today was "I dunno" foods? ____________

Exercise completed today: ______________________________________

______________________________ **Calories burned:** __________

My thoughts and feelings on today's eating and exercise: ____________

____

____

____

DATE ____________ **DAY** ____________

CHECK OFF EACH SERVING YOU EAT OF THE FOLLOWING:
GRAINS (STARCHES) ☐ ☐ ☐ ☐ ☐ ☐ ☐ ☐
FRUITS AND VEGETABLES ☐ ☐ ☐ ☐ ☐
HIGH-CALCIUM FOODS ☐ ☐ ☐
LEAN MEATS, POULTRY, AND EGGS ☐ ☐
FISH ☐ ☐
LEGUMES, NUTS, AND SEEDS ☐ ☐
FAT ☐ ☐
WATER ☐ ☐ ☐ ☐ ☐ ☐ ☐ ☐

Record any foods that don't fit into the above categories and any "I dunno" foods:

FOOD	CALORIES
	Total:

What percentage of your food today was "I dunno" foods?____________

Exercise completed today: ____________________________________

____________________________________ **Calories burned:** __________

My thoughts and feelings on today's eating and exercise: ____________

____

____

____

DATE ________ **DAY** ________

CHECK OFF EACH SERVING YOU EAT OF THE FOLLOWING:
GRAINS (STARCHES) ☐ ☐ ☐ ☐ ☐ ☐ ☐ ☐
FRUITS AND VEGETABLES ☐ ☐ ☐ ☐ ☐
HIGH-CALCIUM FOODS ☐ ☐ ☐
LEAN MEATS, POULTRY, AND EGGS ☐ ☐
FISH ☐ ☐
LEGUMES, NUTS, AND SEEDS ☐ ☐
FAT ☐ ☐
WATER ☐ ☐ ☐ ☐ ☐ ☐ ☐ ☐

Record any foods that don't fit into the above categories and any "I dunno" foods:

FOOD	CALORIES
	Total:

What percentage of your food today was "I dunno" foods? ____________

Exercise completed today: ________________________________

________________________________ **Calories burned:** ________

My thoughts and feelings on today's eating and exercise: ____________

____

____

____

DATE ________ DAY ________

CHECK OFF EACH SERVING YOU EAT OF THE FOLLOWING:
GRAINS (STARCHES) ☐ ☐ ☐ ☐ ☐ ☐ ☐ ☐
FRUITS AND VEGETABLES ☐ ☐ ☐ ☐ ☐
HIGH-CALCIUM FOODS ☐ ☐ ☐
LEAN MEATS, POULTRY, AND EGGS ☐ ☐
FISH ☐ ☐
LEGUMES, NUTS, AND SEEDS ☐ ☐
FAT ☐ ☐
WATER ☐ ☐ ☐ ☐ ☐ ☐ ☐ ☐

Record any foods that don't fit into the above categories and any "I dunno" foods:

FOOD	CALORIES
	Total:

What percentage of your food today was "I dunno" foods? ________

Exercise completed today: ________________________

________________________ **Calories burned:** ________

My thoughts and feelings on today's eating and exercise: ________

____

____

____

DATE ____________ **DAY** ____________

CHECK OFF EACH SERVING YOU EAT OF THE FOLLOWING:
GRAINS (STARCHES) ☐ ☐ ☐ ☐ ☐ ☐ ☐ ☐
FRUITS AND VEGETABLES ☐ ☐ ☐ ☐ ☐
HIGH-CALCIUM FOODS ☐ ☐ ☐
LEAN MEATS, POULTRY, AND EGGS ☐ ☐
FISH ☐ ☐
LEGUMES, NUTS, AND SEEDS ☐ ☐
FAT ☐ ☐
WATER ☐ ☐ ☐ ☐ ☐ ☐ ☐ ☐

Record any foods that don't fit into the above categories and any "I dunno" foods:

FOOD	CALORIES
	Total:

What percentage of your food today was "I dunno" foods? ____________

Exercise completed today: ____________________________________

____________________________________ **Calories burned:** ____________

My thoughts and feelings on today's eating and exercise: ____________

____

____

____

DATE ________ **DAY** ________

CHECK OFF EACH SERVING YOU EAT OF THE FOLLOWING:
GRAINS (STARCHES) ☐ ☐ ☐ ☐ ☐ ☐ ☐ ☐
FRUITS AND VEGETABLES ☐ ☐ ☐ ☐ ☐
HIGH-CALCIUM FOODS ☐ ☐ ☐
LEAN MEATS, POULTRY, AND EGGS ☐ ☐
FISH ☐ ☐
LEGUMES, NUTS, AND SEEDS ☐ ☐
FAT ☐ ☐
WATER ☐ ☐ ☐ ☐ ☐ ☐ ☐ ☐

Record any foods that don't fit into the above categories and any "I dunno" foods:

FOOD	CALORIES
	Total:

What percentage of your food today was "I dunno" foods? ________

Exercise completed today: ________

________ **Calories burned:** ________

My thoughts and feelings on today's eating and exercise: ________

____

____

____

DATE ____________ **DAY** ____________

CHECK OFF EACH SERVING YOU EAT OF THE FOLLOWING:
GRAINS (STARCHES) ☐ ☐ ☐ ☐ ☐ ☐ ☐ ☐
FRUITS AND VEGETABLES ☐ ☐ ☐ ☐ ☐
HIGH-CALCIUM FOODS ☐ ☐ ☐
LEAN MEATS, POULTRY, AND EGGS ☐ ☐
FISH ☐ ☐
LEGUMES, NUTS, AND SEEDS ☐ ☐
FAT ☐ ☐
WATER ☐ ☐ ☐ ☐ ☐ ☐ ☐ ☐

Record any foods that don't fit into the above categories and any "I dunno" foods:

FOOD	CALORIES
	Total:

What percentage of your food today was "I dunno" foods? ____________

Exercise completed today: ____

____ **Calories burned:** ____________

My thoughts and feelings on today's eating and exercise: ____________

____

____

____

Weekly Review

DATE: _________ DAY: ________

WEEK-ENDING WEIGHT: ______ WEIGHT CHANGE THIS WEEK: ______

Diet Danger Zones encountered: ______________________________

____

____

____

Most helpful tools used: ____________________________________

____

____

____

Least helpful tools used: ___________________________________

____

____

____

Patterns I noticed this week: ________________________________

____

____

____

This week I learned that: ___________________________________

____

____

____

Trends that I noticed this week with my portion control and extra "I dunno" foods: ____

____

____

____

WEEK 4

PORTION-CONTROL JOURNAL

DATE: ________ DAY: ________ WEEK-BEGINNING WEIGHT: ________

WEIGHT-LOSS TOOLS TO TRY THIS WEEK:

FOOD TOOL: Why not have a glass of warm milk before you go to bed? It will increase your calcium, fill you up, and maybe even help you sleep.

MOOD TOOL: Are your weight struggles getting you down on yourself? Boost your mood by thinking of all the things you like about yourself: your beautiful nails, your ready smile, your circle of friends. Give yourself a pat on the back for all the great parts of you.

MOVE TOOL: Try yoga. It has so many benefits: It will reduce your stress, improve your flexibility, tone your muscles, and help you lose weight!

BEHAVIOR TOOL: Try waiting before diving into your meal. Be the last to start eating. Delay for a minute or two. Focus. Then start.

Anticipated Diet Danger Zones for this week:

____

Strategies to combat them:

____

____

Goals for the week:

____

____

Calories to burn each day with exercise: ________

MOTIVATIONAL THOUGHT FOR THE WEEK:

When you're truly seeing, there's no failure, only insight.

—Cathy Nonas, R.D.

DATE ______ DAY ______

CHECK OFF EACH SERVING YOU EAT OF THE FOLLOWING:
GRAINS (STARCHES) ☐ ☐ ☐ ☐ ☐ ☐ ☐ ☐
FRUITS AND VEGETABLES ☐ ☐ ☐ ☐ ☐
HIGH-CALCIUM FOODS ☐ ☐ ☐
LEAN MEATS, POULTRY, AND EGGS ☐ ☐
FISH ☐ ☐
LEGUMES, NUTS, AND SEEDS ☐ ☐
FAT ☐ ☐
WATER ☐ ☐ ☐ ☐ ☐ ☐ ☐ ☐

Record any foods that don't fit into the above categories and any "I dunno" foods:

FOOD	CALORIES
	Total:

What percentage of your food today was "I dunno" foods? ______

Exercise completed today: ______

______ **Calories burned:** ______

My thoughts and feelings on today's eating and exercise: ______

______

______

______

DATE ________ **DAY** ________

CHECK OFF EACH SERVING YOU EAT OF THE FOLLOWING:
GRAINS (STARCHES) ☐ ☐ ☐ ☐ ☐ ☐ ☐ ☐
FRUITS AND VEGETABLES ☐ ☐ ☐ ☐ ☐
HIGH-CALCIUM FOODS ☐ ☐ ☐
LEAN MEATS, POULTRY, AND EGGS ☐ ☐
FISH ☐ ☐
LEGUMES, NUTS, AND SEEDS ☐ ☐
FAT ☐ ☐
WATER ☐ ☐ ☐ ☐ ☐ ☐ ☐ ☐

Record any foods that don't fit into the above categories and any "I dunno" foods:

FOOD	CALORIES
	Total:

What percentage of your food today was "I dunno" foods?________

Exercise completed today: ________

________ **Calories burned:** ________

My thoughts and feelings on today's eating and exercise: ________

____

____

____

DATE ____________ **DAY** ____________

CHECK OFF EACH SERVING YOU EAT OF THE FOLLOWING:
GRAINS (STARCHES) ☐ ☐ ☐ ☐ ☐ ☐ ☐ ☐
FRUITS AND VEGETABLES ☐ ☐ ☐ ☐ ☐
HIGH-CALCIUM FOODS ☐ ☐ ☐
LEAN MEATS, POULTRY, AND EGGS ☐ ☐
FISH ☐ ☐
LEGUMES, NUTS, AND SEEDS ☐ ☐
FAT ☐ ☐
WATER ☐ ☐ ☐ ☐ ☐ ☐ ☐ ☐

Record any foods that don't fit into the above categories and any "I dunno" foods:

FOOD	CALORIES
	Total:

What percentage of your food today was "I dunno" foods?____________

Exercise completed today: ____________________________________

____________________________________ **Calories burned:** __________

My thoughts and feelings on today's eating and exercise: __________

____

____

____

DATE ____________ **DAY** ____________

CHECK OFF EACH SERVING YOU EAT OF THE FOLLOWING:
GRAINS (STARCHES) ☐ ☐ ☐ ☐ ☐ ☐ ☐ ☐
FRUITS AND VEGETABLES ☐ ☐ ☐ ☐ ☐
HIGH-CALCIUM FOODS ☐ ☐ ☐
LEAN MEATS, POULTRY, AND EGGS ☐ ☐
FISH ☐ ☐
LEGUMES, NUTS, AND SEEDS ☐ ☐
FAT ☐ ☐
WATER ☐ ☐ ☐ ☐ ☐ ☐ ☐ ☐

Record any foods that don't fit into the above categories and any "I dunno" foods:

FOOD	CALORIES
	Total:

What percentage of your food today was "I dunno" foods? ____________

Exercise completed today: ____

____ **Calories burned:** ____________

My thoughts and feelings on today's eating and exercise: ____________

____

____

____

DATE ______ DAY ______

CHECK OFF EACH SERVING YOU EAT OF THE FOLLOWING:
GRAINS (STARCHES) ☐ ☐ ☐ ☐ ☐ ☐ ☐ ☐
FRUITS AND VEGETABLES ☐ ☐ ☐ ☐ ☐
HIGH-CALCIUM FOODS ☐ ☐ ☐
LEAN MEATS, POULTRY, AND EGGS ☐ ☐
FISH ☐ ☐
LEGUMES, NUTS, AND SEEDS ☐ ☐
FAT ☐ ☐
WATER ☐ ☐ ☐ ☐ ☐ ☐ ☐ ☐

Record any foods that don't fit into the above categories and any "I dunno" foods:

FOOD	CALORIES
	Total:

What percentage of your food today was "I dunno" foods? ______

Exercise completed today: ______

______ **Calories burned:** ______

My thoughts and feelings on today's eating and exercise: ______

______

______

______

DATE ____________ DAY ____________

CHECK OFF EACH SERVING YOU EAT OF THE FOLLOWING:
GRAINS (STARCHES) ☐ ☐ ☐ ☐ ☐ ☐ ☐ ☐
FRUITS AND VEGETABLES ☐ ☐ ☐ ☐ ☐
HIGH-CALCIUM FOODS ☐ ☐ ☐
LEAN MEATS, POULTRY, AND EGGS ☐ ☐
FISH ☐ ☐
LEGUMES, NUTS, AND SEEDS ☐ ☐
FAT ☐ ☐
WATER ☐ ☐ ☐ ☐ ☐ ☐ ☐ ☐

Record any foods that don't fit into the above categories and any "I dunno" foods:

FOOD	CALORIES
	Total:

What percentage of your food today was "I dunno" foods? ____________

Exercise completed today: ____________________________________

____________________________________ **Calories burned:** ____________

My thoughts and feelings on today's eating and exercise: ____________

____

____

____

DATE ______________ **DAY** ______________

CHECK OFF EACH SERVING YOU EAT OF THE FOLLOWING:
GRAINS (STARCHES) ☐ ☐ ☐ ☐ ☐ ☐ ☐ ☐
FRUITS AND VEGETABLES ☐ ☐ ☐ ☐ ☐
HIGH-CALCIUM FOODS ☐ ☐ ☐
LEAN MEATS, POULTRY, AND EGGS ☐ ☐
FISH ☐ ☐
LEGUMES, NUTS, AND SEEDS ☐ ☐
FAT ☐ ☐
WATER ☐ ☐ ☐ ☐ ☐ ☐ ☐ ☐

Record any foods that don't fit into the above categories and any "I dunno" foods:

FOOD	CALORIES
	Total:

What percentage of your food today was "I dunno" foods? ______________

Exercise completed today: ______________________________

______________________________ **Calories burned:** ______________

My thoughts and feelings on today's eating and exercise: ______________

____

____

____

Weekly Review

DATE: ________ DAY: ________

WEEK-ENDING WEIGHT: _____ WEIGHT CHANGE THIS WEEK: _____

Diet Danger Zones encountered: ____________________________

____

____

____

Most helpful tools used: ____________________________

____

____

____

Least helpful tools used: ____________________________

____

____

____

Patterns I noticed this week: ____________________________

____

____

____

This week I learned that: ____________________________

____

____

____

Trends that I noticed this week with my portion control and extra "I dunno" foods: ____________________________

____

____

____

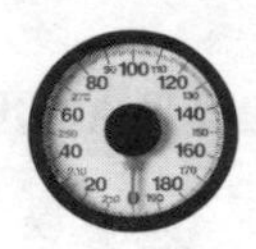

The Overeating Journal

If you're a fairly controlled eater but occasionally "lose it," this journal asks you to record only those times when you feel you've overeaten or your eating has gotten out of control. You may have 3 such times in a week or 3 in one day. The episode could last for a few hours or an entire day. Just having your journal with you may discourage you from impulsive overeating. It can also help you see a destructive pattern that's easier to change than you realized.

This journal has three columns. Column one is for food, column two is for how the food was eaten, and column three is for your hand-to-mouth behavior. (So named because it's the act of moving the hand to the mouth—not the food itself—that's important.) The goal: more "nos" in column three.

Photocopy this one-page journal. Tuck one copy into your wallet and tape another to your fridge door. That way, you'll have it if you suddenly fall prey to an overeating "emergency." Use it for all overeating, including trips to the kitchen after dinner.

DATE *11/5/02* **DAY** *23*

OVEREATING JOURNAL
SAMPLE PAGE

Situation: *After dinner*

Companions: *Mother, father, sister*

Record everything you ate:

FOOD	HOW EATEN	HAND TO MOUTH?
Cup of hot cocoa	*Watching TV*	*No*
Bag of popcorn	*Watching TV*	*Yes*
Cheese and crackers	*Standing at counter*	*Yes*
Bowl of ice cream	*While on phone*	*Yes*

DATE ____________ **DAY** ____________

Situation: ______________________________

Companions: ______________________________

Record everything you ate:

FOOD	HOW EATEN	HAND TO MOUTH?

Situation: ______________________________

Companions: ______________________________

Record everything you ate:

FOOD	HOW EATEN	HAND TO MOUTH?

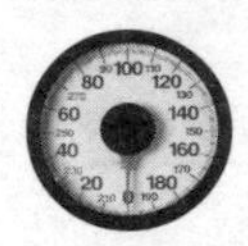

The Social-Butterfly Journal

If dining out is your most formidable Diet Danger Zone, this journal asks that you record what you're eating *as you eat it*, not after you leave the restaurant. Yes, to use this diary, you need to commit to writing in front of people or going to the restroom to record that you've just eaten your second garlic breadstick. But it's worth it: Journaling may keep you from taking a third.

Photocopy page 152 and slip it into your wallet or bag. (You can always borrow a pen if you need to.)

Periodically, look back at your journal entries and look for patterns. For example, do you eat more when you're with your spouse or with your friends? Are there certain restaurants where you lose all control? Are there others where you're able to make excellent food choices?

Unlike the other journals, which ask you to record your exercise or your inner thoughts, this one asks you to record how you feel about your appearance. (After all, you *are* a social butterfly.) Think about whether you feel good about your appearance and so are sticking to your program or whether you feel insecure about how you look, which is causing you to hit the mozzarella sticks more than you want to.

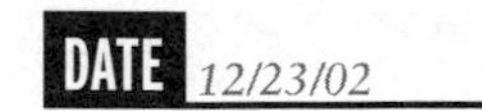 *12/23/02* 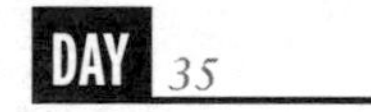 *35*

SAMPLE PAGE

Event: *Company holiday dinner dance*

Companions: *Michael, Molly and Jeff, Jennifer and Frank, Carol and Tim*

Appearance: *Great! I fit into the skinny black dress I found at Macy's*

Record everything you ate:

FOOD	HAPPY?	BETTER OPTIONS?
BEVERAGES *3 glasses white wine*	*Only with the first*	*Only have one glass*
APPETIZERS *4 boiled shrimp* *4 mini fried egg rolls*	*Yes* *No*	 *4 more shrimp*
BREAD *1 roll with butter*	*No*	*Roll without butter*
ENTRÉE *Flounder stuffed with crabmeat* *½ cup broccoli*	*Yes, since it was the healthiest of three choices.* *Yes*	
DESSERT *Fruit cup*	*Yes*	

DATE ____________ DAY ____________

Event: ____

____

Companions: ____

____

Appearance: ____

____

Record everything you ate:

FOOD	HAPPY?	BETTER OPTIONS?
BEVERAGES		
APPETIZERS		
BREAD		
ENTRÉE		
DESSERT		

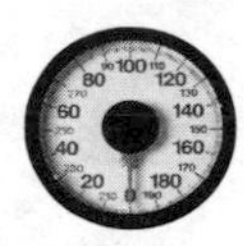

The Fullness Journal

For some people, there's no such thing as being a "little" full. By the time they feel full, they're in actual physical discomfort. If this sounds like you, try this journal.

Photocopy this one-page journal. You'll fill this out every few months. Think about times when you've felt stuffed, too full, and comfortable. Choose the adjectives that describe how you felt each time, then record your physical sensations. For "Stuffed," do you feel tired? Nauseated? Bloated? Describe a situation in which you've felt this way before, such as a company party or dinner out with friends.

For "Too Full," describe how you feel when you are too full but not quite stuffed. Describe a past eating situation that caused you to feel this way.

In the "Comfortable" column, describe how you feel when you have eaten just enough. How many physical symptoms can you name? None, you say? You're not alone. Most people have a hard time trying to define physical symptoms of having had just enough. Here's how to learn what "full" feels like.

At your next meal, just eat half of your meal. Stop eating, then ask yourself these questions:

1. Do I have to loosen my belt?

2. Do I feel more fatigued?

3. Could I leave the table sooner?

4. Could I have eaten less and been as satisfied?

If the answer is "yes" to any of these, you're too full. Regardless of which column you select, reread your journal entries to remind yourself how good it feels to be comfortably full rather than too full or stuffed.

Another way to use this journal is, after you've finished a meal, put a check mark in the column that describes how you feel.

DATE *12/30/02* **DAY** *42*

FULLNESS JOURNAL
SAMPLE PAGE

RECORD YOUR PHYSICAL SENSATIONS:

STUFFED	TOO FULL	COMFORTABLE
Nauseated	*Uncomfortable*	*Energized*
Bloated	*Displeased and slightly guilty*	*Satisfied*
Clothes are too tight	*Sluggish*	*Could eat more, but not necessary*
Guilty	*Felt as if I wanted to loosen my belt*	*Proud that I left the table before I was too full*
Sleepy	*Tired*	*Just right*

DATE ____________ DAY ____________

RECORD YOUR PHYSICAL SENSATIONS:

STUFFED	TOO FULL	COMFORTABLE

Part 3

THE CHARTS

CALORIES, FAT, AND FIBER FOR MORE THAN 500 FOODS

Put away your calculator. The chart that follows can make it simpler than you may think to keep track of the calories, fat, and fiber in the foods you eat. The best part? No number crunching is necessary (unless you want to do it, of course).

Like most other nutrient counters, this chart divvies up food into categories, from beans to vegetables. In between, you'll find breakfast foods, desserts, snack foods, fish and shellfish, meats, and so forth.

Here's some other information that you'll need to use this chart.

- We've rounded calorie counts to the nearest whole number and fat and fiber values to the nearest tenth of a gram.

- Unless otherwise specified, the foods are commercially prepared.

- While brand names are used in some cases, the nutrient information for many commercially prepared foods (such as frozen entrées) should be viewed as sample values. Expect variations among different brands and read labels carefully.

- There are no fiber listings for animal products, fish, shellfish, fats, oils, and some spreads since those foods contain no fiber.

Also, keep in mind that just about every food you buy has a nutrition information label, so you can just check the labels for the calorie, fat, and fiber numbers.

BEANS, BEAN PRODUCTS, AND OTHER LEGUMES				
FOOD	PORTION	CAL.	FAT (G)	FIBER (G)
Adzuki beans, boiled	½ cup	147	0.1	8.5
Baked beans with pork, canned	½ cup	134	2	6.9
Black beans, boiled	½ cup	114	0.5	7.5
Broad beans (fava beans), boiled	½ cup	94	0.3	4.6
Chickpeas, canned	½ cup	143	1.4	5.6
Chili, vegetarian, canned	1 cup	286	14	11.2
Chili with beans and meat, canned	1 cup	250	11	8
Green peas, boiled	½ cup	67	0.2	2.4
Lentils, boiled	½ cup	114	0.4	7.8
Lima beans, boiled	½ cup	108	0.4	6.6
Refried beans, canned	½ cup	135	1.4	6.7
Snap beans (green beans), boiled	½ cup	22	0.2	2
Soybeans, boiled	½ cup	149	7.7	5
Soybean sprouts, raw	½ cup	45	2.4	0.4
Split peas, boiled	½ cup	116	0.4	8.1
Tempeh	½ cup	165	6.4	0
Tofu, firm, raw	¼ block (3 oz)	118	7.1	1.9

BREADS AND BREAD PRODUCTS				
FOOD	PORTION	CAL.	FAT (G)	FIBER (G)
Bagel, plain or onion	1 (2½ oz)	195	1.1	1.5
Biscuit, baking powder, homemade	1 (1 oz)	103	4.8	0.5
Biscuit, buttermilk, Pillsbury Hungry Jack	1	100	4.5	0
Blueberry muffin, homemade with 2% milk	1 (2 oz)	163	6.2	0
Bran muffin, homemade with wheat bran and 2% milk	1 (2 oz)	161	7	2.6
Breadstick, plain	1 (¼ oz)	25	0.6	0.6
Cinnamon roll, refrigerator, baked, with frosting	1 roll	150	4	1

(continued)

BREADS AND BREAD PRODUCTS (CONT.)

FOOD	PORTION	CAL.	FAT (G)	FIBER (G)
Corn muffin, homemade with 2% milk	1 (2 oz)	180	7	0
Cracked wheat bread	1 slice (1 oz)	65	1	1.3
Croissant	1 (2 oz)	235	12	1.5
English muffin, plain, toasted	1 (2 oz)	133	1	1.5
French, Vienna, or sourdough bread	1 slice (1 oz)	69	0.8	0.7
Italian bread	1 slice (1 oz)	81	1.1	0.9
Pita bread, white	1 (2 oz)	165	0.7	1
Popover, homemade	1 (1½ oz)	90	3.7	0
Pumpernickel bread	1 slice (1 oz)	80	1	1.9
Raisin bread	1 slice (1 oz)	71	1.1	1.1
Roll or bun, homemade with whole milk	1 (1 oz)	112	2.7	0.8
Rye bread	1 slice (1 oz)	83	1.1	2
Spoon bread, homemade with vegetable shortening	1 cup	468	27.4	0
Wheat bread, reduced-calorie	1 slice (1 oz)	46	0.5	2.6
White bread, soft crumb	1 slice (1 oz)	67	0.9	0.6
Zwieback rusks	5 pieces (1 oz)	149	3.4	0.9

BREAKFAST FOODS

FOOD	PORTION	CAL.	FAT (G)	FIBER (G)
Cold Cereals				
Cheerios with fat-free milk	1 cup with ½ cup milk	150	2	3
Cracklin' Oat Bran with fat-free milk	¾ cup with ½ cup milk	270	8	5
Granola without raisins, low-fat, with fat-free milk	½ cup with ½ cup milk	250	3	3.2
Kellogg's Frosted Flakes with fat-free milk	¾ cup with ½ cup milk	160	0	1
Raisin Bran with fat-free milk	1 cup with ½ cup milk	210	1	8

FOOD	PORTION	CAL.	FAT (G)	FIBER (G)
Shredded Wheat without milk	2 biscuits	160	0.5	6
Trix with fat-free milk	1 cup with ½ cup milk	160	1.5	0
Hot Cereals				
Cream of Rice, cooked	¾ cup	95	0.2	0.2
Cream of Wheat, quick-cooking, cooked	¾ cup	97	0.4	1
Farina, enriched, cooked	¾ cup	88	0.2	2.5
Oatmeal, cooked	¾ cup	109	1.8	4
Ralston, cooked	¾ cup	101	0.6	5
Wheatena, cooked	⅓ cup	160	1	5
Others				
Biscuit with egg, cheese, and sausage, frozen	1 (5 oz)	470	30	1
Biscuit with egg and sausage (McDonald's)	1 (6½ oz)	520	35	1
Coffee cake	1 slice (2 oz)	240	12	0.5
Croissant with egg, cheese, and sausage (Burger King)	1 (6 oz)	530	41	0
Danish, cheese (McDonald's)	1 (4 oz)	410	22	0
Doughnut, cream-filled, yeast or raised	1 (3 oz)	307	20.8	0.7
Doughnut, plain, made without yeast	1 (2 oz)	198	10.8	0.8
English muffin with egg, cheese, and Canadian bacon (McDonald's)	1 (5 oz)	290	13	1
French toast, frozen, with low-calorie syrup	2 slices (4 oz total) with 4 Tbsp syrup	340	6	1.3
French toast sticks without butter and syrup (Burger King)	5 (5½ oz total)	500	27	1
Hash browns, frozen, oven-heated	1 patty (2½ oz)	110	6	2

(continued)

BREAKFAST FOODS (CONT.)

FOOD	PORTION	CAL.	FAT (G)	FIBER (G)
Others (cont.)				
Hash browns (McDonald's)	1 patty (2 oz)	130	8	1
Pancakes with 2 pats margarine and syrup (McDonald's)	3 (9 oz total)	560	14	2
Toaster pastry with fruit (Pop-Tart)	1	200	5.3	1
Waffle, frozen, with low-calorie syrup	1 (1¼ oz) with 2 Tbsp syrup	136	2.1	2

CANDY AND SWEETS

FOOD	PORTION	CAL.	FAT (G)	FIBER (G)
Almonds, chocolate-coated	7 (1 oz total)	159	12.2	2.4
Butterscotch	4 pieces	112	1	0
Caramels	3 (1 oz total)	108	2.3	0.3
Chocolate bar, semisweet	1 (1½ oz)	230	13	2
Coconut bar, chocolate-coated	1 (2 oz)	195	11.7	1.7
Fudge, chocolate with nuts, homemade	1 piece (1 oz)	121	4.6	0.4
Fudge, vanilla, homemade	1 piece (1 oz)	105	1.5	0
Hard candy	3 pieces	60	0	0
Marshmallow chicks	5 small	160	0	0
Mints, chocolate-coated	2 (⅓ oz total)	29	1.1	0.2
Peanut brittle	1 piece	180	5	0.8
Peanuts, chocolate-coated	10 (1½ oz total)	208	13.4	1.7
Raisins, chocolate-coated	10 (⅓ oz total)	39	1.5	0.4

CHEESE AND CHEESE PRODUCTS

FOOD	PORTION	CAL.	FAT (G)	FIBER (G)
American				
fat-free	1 slice (¾ oz)	30	0	0
regular	1 oz	106	8.9	0
Blue cheese	1 oz	99	8.1	0

FOOD	PORTION	CAL.	FAT (G)	FIBER (G)
Brie	1 oz	93	7.6	0
Camembert	1 oz	84	6.8	0
Caraway	1 oz	105	8.2	0
Cheddar				
fat-free	1 oz	45	0	0
reduced-fat	1 oz	80	5	0
regular	1 oz	113	9	0
Colby	1 oz	110	9	0
Cottage cheese				
creamed, small or large curd	½ cup	109	4.7	0
1%	½ cup	82	1.2	0
2%	½ cup	101	2.2	0
Cream cheese				
fat-free	2 Tbsp	30	0	0
reduced-fat	2 Tbsp	70	5	0
regular	1 oz	98	10	0
Feta	1 oz	74	6	0
Fondue	¼ cup	151	10.4	0
Gouda	1 oz	100	7.7	0
Gruyère	1 oz	116	9.1	0
Limburger	1 oz	92	7.6	0
Monterey Jack	1 oz	105	8.5	0
Mozzarella				
reduced-fat	1 oz	71	4.5	0
regular	1 oz	79	6.1	0
Muenster				
reduced-fat	1 oz	80	5	0
regular	1 oz	103	8.4	0
Neufchâtel	1 oz	73	6.6	0
Parmesan, grated	1 Tbsp	23	1.5	0
Provolone	1 oz	98	7.5	0

(continued)

CHEESE AND CHEESE PRODUCTS (CONT.)

FOOD	PORTION	CAL.	FAT (G)	FIBER (G)
Ricotta				
reduced-fat	½ cup	171	9.8	0
regular	½ cup	216	16.1	0
Romano, grated	1 Tbsp	19	1.4	0
Soufflé, homemade	1 cup	207	16.2	0
Swiss				
fat-free	1 slice (¾ oz)	30	0	0
regular	1 oz	105	7.7	0
Yogurt cheese, low-fat	1 oz	30	0.6	0
Welsh rarebit, frozen	¼ cup (2 oz)	120	9	0

DESSERTS

FOOD	PORTION	CAL.	FAT (G)	FIBER (G)
Cakes				
Angel food	1 slice (1⁄12 of cake)	73	0.2	0.4
Boston cream	1 slice (⅙ of cake)	232	7.8	1.2
Carrot cake, homemade with cream cheese icing	1 slice (1⁄12 of cake)	484	29.3	1
Cheesecake, frozen	¼ cake (4¼ oz)	350	18	0.4
Devil's food, made from mix with eggs and oil, with 2 Tbsp chocolate icing	1 slice (1⁄12 of cake)	440	21	3
Fruitcake	1 slice (2 oz)	139	3.9	1.5
Pound, made with butter	1 slice (1⁄12 of cake)	110	5.6	0.1
Sponge	1 slice (1⁄12 of cake)	110	1	0.2
White, made from mix with egg whites and oil, with 2 Tbsp reduced-calorie chocolate icing	1 slice (1⁄12 of cake)	370	11	1.1
Yellow with pudding, made from mix with eggs and margarine, with 2 Tbsp chocolate icing	1 slice (1⁄12 of cake)	410	17	1.5

FOOD	PORTION	CAL.	FAT (G)	FIBER (G)
Cookies				
Brownie with nuts, made from mix	1 (3/4 oz)	81	3.7	0.4
Chocolate chip, homemade with margarine	1 (1/2 oz)	78	4.5	0.6
Fig bars	2 (1 oz total)	110	2.5	1.5
Gingersnaps	5 (1 1/4 oz total)	147	3.1	0.8
Ladyfingers	4 (1 1/2 oz total)	158	3.4	0.4
Macaroon, homemade	1 (1 oz)	97	3.1	0.5
Molasses	2 (2 oz total)	274	6.9	0.6
Oatmeal with raisins				
homemade	1 (1/2 oz)	65	2.4	0.5
reduced-fat	2 (1 oz total)	110	2.5	1
Peanut butter, homemade	1 (3/4 oz)	95	4.8	0.5
Sandwich, vanilla with cream filling	4 (2 oz total)	297	13.5	1
Sugar, homemade with margarine	1 (1/2 oz)	66	3.3	0.2
Sugar wafer with cream filling	1 small	18	0.9	0
Vanilla wafers	8 (1 oz total)	150	7	1
Pies				
Apple, fresh	1 slice (1/8 of pie)	302	13.1	2.2
Banana custard, fresh	1 slice (1/8 of pie)	252	10.6	1.5
Blueberry, fresh	1 slice (1/8 of pie)	286	12.7	2.3
Cherry, fresh	1 slice (1/8 of pie)	308	13.3	3
Chocolate meringue, fresh	1 slice (1/8 of pie)	287	13.7	2
Custard, fresh	1 slice (1/8 of pie)	249	12.7	1.5
Lemon meringue, fresh	1 slice (1/8 of pie)	268	10.7	1
Mince, fresh	1 slice (1/8 of pie)	320	13.6	4.2
Pecan, fresh	1 slice (1/8 of pie)	431	23.6	3
Pumpkin, fresh	1 slice (1/8 of pie)	241	12.8	2.3

(continued)

DESSERTS (CONT.)

FOOD	PORTION	CAL.	FAT (G)	FIBER (G)
Pudding				
Chocolate, made from mix with whole milk	½ cup	163	4.6	1.5
Custard, homemade, baked	½ cup	148	6.6	0
Rice, homemade	½ cup	175	4.1	0.1
Tapioca, made from mix with whole milk	½ cup	161	4.1	0
Vanilla, made from mix with 2% milk	½ cup	148	2.4	0
Others				
Eclair	1 (3½ oz)	239	13.6	0.5
Fruit cocktail, canned in light syrup	½ cup	72	0.1	1.4
Gelatin, made from powder	½ cup	80	0.1	0

DIPS AND SNACKS

FOOD	PORTION	CAL.	FAT (G)	FIBER (G)
Dips				
Bacon and horseradish	2 Tbsp	60	5	0
Cheese				
low-fat	2 Tbsp	80	3	0
regular	2 Tbsp	90	7	0
Clam	2 Tbsp	50	4.5	0
Hummus	⅓ cup	140	6.9	5
Onion				
low-fat	2 Tbsp	30	0	0
regular	2 Tbsp	60	5	0
Ranch	2 Tbsp	140	14	0
Salsa	2 Tbsp	10	0	0.5
Snacks				
Caramel corn	½ cup	140	4	1
Cereal mix	¾ cup	130	5	1.5
Cheez Doodles	17 (1 oz total)	150	8	0

FOOD	PORTION	CAL.	FAT (G)	FIBER (G)
Corn chips	30 small (1 oz total)	155	9.1	1
Cracker Jacks	1 box	150	3	1.3
Crackers				
butter-flavored	4 (½ oz total)	64	2.5	0.3
cheese	4 round (½ oz total)	67	3	0.3
cheese and peanut butter	2 (½ oz total)	69	3.4	0.4
wheat	7 (½ oz total)	61	1.8	0.6
Crispbread, rye	1 slice	35	0	1.5
Fruit rolls	2	110	1	0.6
Graham crackers	1 (½ oz)	55	1.3	0.4
Granola bar, chocolate chip	1 (1 oz)	120	3.5	1
Granola bar, chocolate chip, low-fat	1 (1 oz)	110	2	1
Melba toast	3 pieces (½ oz total)	55	0.5	0.9
Popcorn				
air-popped, plain	1 cup	31	0.3	1.2
buttered	1 cup	41	2	1
microwave, butter-flavored	1 bag (13 cups)	150	10	4
Potato chips				
fat-free	30 (1 oz total)	110	0	2
regular	10 (¾ oz total)	105	7.1	1
Potato sticks	1 oz	148	9.8	1
Pretzels				
baked	16 (1 oz total)	120	2.5	0.8
Dutch-type	2 large (1 oz total)	125	1.4	0.9
whole wheat	1 oz	102	0.7	2.2
Rice cakes, flavored	1 (½ oz)	50	0	0.8
Saltine crackers	5 (½ oz total)	61	1.7	0.4
Sesame sticks	30 pieces (1 oz total)	170	12	0.8

(continued)

DIPS AND SNACKS (CONT.)

FOOD	PORTION	CAL.	FAT (G)	FIBER (G)
Snacks (cont.)				
Toffee corn (popcorn and peanuts)	⅔ cup (1 oz)	140	4	1.1
Tortilla chips, plain	13 (1 oz total)	140	6	1.8

DRESSINGS

FOOD	PORTION	CAL.	FAT (G)	FIBER (G)
Blue cheese				
fat-free	2 Tbsp	35	0	0
low-fat	2 Tbsp	80	8	0
regular	2 Tbsp	170	17	0
Caesar				
low-fat	2 Tbsp	70	6	0
regular	2 Tbsp	170	18	0
French				
fat-free	2 Tbsp	50	0	0
low-fat	2 Tbsp	50	3	0
regular	2 Tbsp	120	12	0
Garlic, creamy				
fat-free	2 Tbsp	40	0	0
regular	2 Tbsp	140	13	0
Honey Dijon				
fat-free	2 Tbsp	50	0	0
regular	2 Tbsp	130	10	0
Italian				
fat-free	2 Tbsp	15	0	0
low-fat	2 Tbsp	15	0.5	0
regular	2 Tbsp	100	10	0
Italian, creamy				
low-fat	2 Tbsp	50	5	0
regular	2 Tbsp	110	11	0
Oil and vinegar				
low-fat	2 Tbsp	60	5	0
regular	2 Tbsp	110	11	0

FOOD	PORTION	CAL.	FAT (G)	FIBER (G)
Oil and vinegar, imitation, fat-free	2 Tbsp	15	0	0
Ranch				
fat-free	2 Tbsp	45	0	0
low-fat	2 Tbsp	80	7	0
regular	2 Tbsp	140	14	0
Russian	2 Tbsp	110	6	0
Sweet-and-sour	2 Tbsp	150	13	0
Thousand Island				
fat-free	2 Tbsp	35	0	0
low-fat	2 Tbsp	45	1	0
regular	2 Tbsp	110	10	0

EGGS AND EGG SUBSTITUTE

FOOD	PORTION	CAL.	FAT (G)	FIBER (G)
Egg				
fried with margarine	1 large	92	6.9	0
hard-boiled	1 large	78	5.3	0
scrambled with butter and whole milk	1 large	95	7.1	0
Egg substitute				
frozen	¼ cup	96	6.7	0
liquid	¼ cup	53	2.1	0
Egg white	1 large	16	Trace	0
Egg yolk	1 large	59	5.1	0
Quiche				
Lorraine	1 slice (6¼ oz)	600	48	0
spinach, frozen	1 (6 oz)	480	32	0.4

FAST FOODS

FOOD	PORTION	CAL.	FAT (G)	FIBER (G)
Arby's				
Baked potato with broccoli and cheese	1	540	17.9	7
Roast beef on bun	1	330	14	2

(continued)

FAST FOODS (CONT.)

FOOD	PORTION	CAL.	FAT (G)	FIBER (G)
Arby's (cont.)				
Submarine, Italian (cold cuts)	1	671	38.8	3
Submarine, turkey	1	630	37	2
Burger King				
Cheeseburger with condiments on bun	1	380	13	1
Double cheeseburger with condiments on bun	1	600	36	1
Onion rings, breaded	1 order	310	14	5
Pie, apple	1	310	15	2
KFC				
Chicken breast, fried	1	360	20	1
Chicken breast and wing quarter, roasted, without skin	1	199	5.9	0
Chicken nuggets without sauce	6	284	18	0
McDonald's				
Fish, breaded, with tartar sauce on bun	1	360	16	1
French fries	1 large	450	22	5
Hamburger with condiments on bun	1	270	9	2
Shake, chocolate	1 small	350	6	1
Shake, vanilla	1 small	310	5	0
Taco Bell				
Burrito, bean	1	391	12	12
Burrito, supreme	1	440	18	8
Nachos	1 order	310	18	3
Taco, beef	1	170	10	1
Wendy's				
Baked potato with cheese and bacon	1	530	18	7
Baked potato with chili and cheese	1	610	24	9

FOOD	PORTION	CAL.	FAT (G)	FIBER (G)
Baked potato with sour cream and chives	1	380	6	8
Chicken, breaded, with mayonnaise, lettuce, and tomato on bun	1	450	20	2
Garden salad with 2 Tbsp reduced-fat, reduced-calorie Italian dressing	1	150	9	4
Taco salad with small chili and 1 packet sour cream	1	830	42	11

FATS, OILS, AND SPREADS

FOOD	PORTION	CAL.	FAT (G)	FIBER (G)
Fats				
Chicken	1 Tbsp	115	12.8	0
Lard	1 Tbsp	115	12.8	0
Shortening	1 Tbsp	113	12.8	0
Oils				
Almond	1 Tbsp	120	13.6	0
Avocado	1 Tbsp	124	14	0
Canola	1 Tbsp	124	14	0
Coconut	1 Tbsp	120	13.6	0
Corn	1 Tbsp	120	13.6	0
Cottonseed	1 Tbsp	120	13.6	0
Grapeseed	1 Tbsp	120	13.6	0
Olive	1 Tbsp	119	13.5	0
Palm	1 Tbsp	120	13.6	0
Peanut	1 Tbsp	119	13.5	0
Safflower	1 Tbsp	120	13.6	0
Sesame	1 Tbsp	120	13.6	0
Soybean	1 Tbsp	120	13.6	0
Sunflower	1 Tbsp	120	13.6	0
Walnut	1 Tbsp	120	13.6	0

(continued)

FATS, OILS, AND SPREADS (CONT.)

FOOD	PORTION	CAL.	FAT (G)	FIBER (G)
Spreads				
Almond butter, unsalted	1 Tbsp	101	9.5	0.6
Apple butter	1 Tbsp	33	0.1	0.3
Butter, salted, unsalted stick, or whipped	1 Tbsp	102	11.5	0
Butter blend, made with butter and vegetable oil	1 Tbsp	50	6	0
Margarine				
squeeze	1 Tbsp	80	9	0
stick, reduced-fat	1 Tbsp	60	6	0
stick, regular	1 Tbsp	100	11	0
tub, reduced-fat	1 Tbsp	45	4.5	0
tub, regular	1 Tbsp	100	11	0
Mayonnaise				
low-fat	1 Tbsp	25	1	0
reduced-fat	1 Tbsp	50	5	0
regular	1 Tbsp	100	11	0
Peanut butter, smooth	2 Tbsp	188	16	1.9

FISH AND SHELLFISH

FOOD	PORTION	CAL.	FAT (G)	FIBER (G)
Fish				
Anchovies, canned in olive oil	5 (3/4 oz total)	42	1.9	0
Bass, striped, baked or broiled	3 oz	124	4	0
Bluefish, cooked, dry heat	3 oz	135	4.6	0
Carp, broiled, baked, or microwaved	3 oz	138	6.1	0
Catfish, broiled, baked, or microwaved	3 oz	89	2.4	0
Caviar, black or red	1 Tbsp	40	2.9	0
Cod, Atlantic, broiled, baked, or microwaved	3 oz	89	0.7	0

FOOD	PORTION	CAL.	FAT (G)	FIBER (G)
Eel, broiled, baked, or microwaved	3 oz	201	12.7	0
Flounder, broiled, baked, or microwaved	3 oz	99	1.3	0
Grouper, broiled, baked, or microwaved	3 oz	100	1.1	0
Haddock, broiled, baked, or microwaved	3 oz	95	0.8	0
Halibut, broiled, baked, or microwaved	3 oz	119	2.5	0
Herring, kippered	1 fillet (1½ oz)	87	5	0
Mackerel, Atlantic, broiled, baked, or microwaved	3 oz	223	15.1	0
Monkfish, cooked, dry heat	3 oz	82	1.6	0
Ocean perch, Atlantic, broiled, baked, or microwaved	3 oz	103	1.8	0
Orange roughy, broiled, baked, or microwaved	3 oz	75	0.8	0
Pollack, broiled, baked, or microwaved	3 oz	96	1	0
Pompano, Florida, broiled, baked, or microwaved	3 oz	179	10.3	0
Salmon				
pink, canned, with bones and liquid	3 oz	118	5.1	0
sockeye, fresh, broiled, baked, or microwaved	3 oz	184	9.3	0
Sardines, Atlantic, canned in oil, drained, with bones	2 (1 oz total)	50	2.8	0
Smelt, rainbow, broiled, baked, or microwaved	3 oz	105	2.6	0
Snapper, mixed species, broiled, baked, or microwaved	3 oz	109	1.5	0
Sole, broiled, baked, or microwaved	3 oz	99	1.3	0
Surimi, uncooked	3 oz	84	0.7	0

(continued)

FISH AND SHELLFISH (CONT.)

FOOD	PORTION	CAL.	FAT (G)	FIBER (G)
Fish (cont.)				
Swordfish, broiled, baked, or microwaved	3 oz	132	4.4	0
Trout, rainbow, broiled, baked, or microwaved	3 oz	128	3.7	0
Tuna, fresh, broiled, baked, or microwaved	3 oz	156	5.3	0
Tuna, light meat, canned in water	3 oz	99	0.7	0
Tuna salad, prepared with mayonnaise	3 oz	159	7.9	0
Turbot, European, uncooked	3 oz	81	2.5	0
Whitefish, mixed species, smoked	3 oz	92	0.8	0
Shellfish				
Clams, breaded and fried	20 small (6¾ oz total)	380	21	0
Clams, steamed	20 small (3 oz)	133	1.8	0
Crab, Alaskan king, steamed	3 oz	82	1.3	0
Crab, soft-shell, fried	1 (4½ oz)	334	17.9	0
Crayfish (crawfish), steamed	3 oz	97	1.2	0
Lobster, boiled, poached, or steamed	3 oz	83	0.5	0
Lobster salad, prepared with mayonnaise	½ cup	286	16.6	0
Mussels, blue, boiled, poached, or steamed	3 oz	146	3.8	0
Oysters, Eastern, breaded and fried	6 medium (3 oz total)	173	11.1	0
Oysters, Eastern, steamed	6 medium (1½ oz total)	57	2.1	0
Scallops, breaded and fried	2 large (1 oz total)	67	3.4	0
Shrimp, breaded and fried	3 oz	206	10.4	0.6
Shrimp, steamed	3 oz	84	0.9	0

FRUITS AND FRUIT JUICES				
FOOD	**PORTION**	**CAL.**	**FAT (G)**	**FIBER (G)**
Apple, raw, with skin	1	81	0.5	3.7
Apple juice, unsweetened, canned or bottled	1 cup	117	0.3	0.3
Avocado	½	162	15.4	2.5
Cherries, sweet, without pits	1 cup	104	1.4	3.3
Figs, dried	3 (2 oz total)	145	0.7	5.2
Grapefruit, pink	½	37	0.1	1.4
Grapes, green or red	1 cup	114	0.9	1.6
Orange juice, frozen, from concentrate	1 cup	112	0.2	0.5
Peach, raw	1	37	0.1	1.7
Pears, canned in light syrup	½ cup	72	0.04	2.5
Raisins, seedless	½ cup	218	0.3	2.9
Strawberries	1 cup	45	0.6	3.4

GRAINS				
FOOD	**PORTION**	**CAL.**	**FAT (G)**	**FIBER (G)**
Barley, pearled, cooked	½ cup	97	0.4	3
Bran				
oat, raw	2 Tbsp	29	0.8	1.8
rice, raw	2 Tbsp	33	2.2	3
wheat, raw	2 Tbsp	15	0.3	3
Buckwheat groats, cooked	½ cup	91	0.6	2.2
Bulgur wheat, cooked	½ cup	76	0.2	4.1
Corn grits, white or yellow, cooked	½ cup	73	0.2	0.2
Cornmeal, whole grain, white or yellow, raw	¼ cup	109	1.1	2.2
Couscous, cooked	½ cup	101	0.1	1.3
Hominy, white or yellow, canned, raw	½ cup	58	0.7	2
Millet, cooked	½ cup	143	1.2	2.3
Quinoa, raw	¼ cup	159	2.5	2.5

(continued)

GRAINS (CONT.)

FOOD	PORTION	CAL.	FAT (G)	FIBER (G)
Rice				
brown, cooked	½ cup	109	0.9	1.8
white				
enriched, cooked	½ cup	133	0.3	0.4
instant, cooked	½ cup	80	0.1	0.5
wild, cooked	½ cup	83	0.3	1.5
Rye, raw	¼ cup	141	1.1	6.1
Wheat germ, toasted	¼ cup	108	3	3.7

GRAVIES AND SAUCES

FOOD	PORTION	CAL.	FAT (G)	FIBER (G)
Gravies				
Au jus, canned	¼ cup	10	0.1	0
Beef, canned	¼ cup	31	1.4	0.2
Brown, dry mix, prepared	¼ cup	19	0.4	0.4
Chicken, canned	¼ cup	47	3.4	0.2
Mushroom, canned	¼ cup	30	1.6	0.2
Onion, dry mix, prepared	¼ cup	20	0.2	0.4
Turkey, canned	¼ cup	30	1.3	0.2
Sauces				
Alfredo, canned	½ cup	310	27	0
Barbecue, bottled	¼ cup	47	1.1	0.3
Curry, dry mix, made with milk	¼ cup	67	3.7	0
Hollandaise, dry mix, made with milk and butter	¼ cup	176	17.1	0.1
Marinara, canned	½ cup	71	2.6	2
Soy, tamari, bottled	1 Tbsp	11	0.1	0.1
Spaghetti, canned	½ cup	71	2.6	2
Sweet-and-sour, dry mix, made with water and vinegar	¼ cup	74	0.02	0.4
Teriyaki, bottled	¼ cup	60	0	0
Tomato, canned	1 cup	74	0.4	3.4

FOOD	PORTION	CAL.	FAT (G)	FIBER (G)
White				
dry mix, made with milk	¼ cup	60	3.4	0.1
homemade	¼ cup	101	7.8	0.1

ICE CREAM AND FROZEN TREATS

FOOD	PORTION	CAL.	FAT (G)	FIBER (G)
Frozen yogurt, vanilla				
fat-free	½ cup	110	0	0
regular	½ cup	110	1.5	0
Fruit ice	1 cup	247	0	0
Fruit juice bar	1 (1¾ oz)	42	0	0
Ice cream, soft-serve, chocolate or vanilla, on cone	1 (5 oz)	230	7	0.1
Ice cream, vanilla				
reduced-fat	½ cup	130	4.5	0
regular	½ cup	170	10	0
Ice cream sundae, chocolate	1 (6 oz)	300	7	0
Ice milk, soft-serve, vanilla	½ cup	112	2.3	0
Sherbet, orange	½ cup	135	1.9	0
Tofutti, all flavors	½ cup	217	12	0

MEATS

FOOD	PORTION	CAL.	FAT (G)	FIBER (G)
Beef				
Brisket, lean, braised	3 oz	206	10.9	0
Corned beef hash, canned	1 cup	398	24.9	0
Ground, broiled				
extra-lean	3 oz	225	13.4	0
lean	3 oz	238	15	0
regular	3 oz	248	16.5	0
Liver, braised	3 oz	137	4.2	0
Meat loaf	3 oz	170	11.2	0

(continued)

MEATS (CONT.)

FOOD	PORTION	CAL.	FAT (G)	FIBER (G)
Beef (cont.)				
Roast				
bottom round, lean, braised	3 oz	178	7	0
pot, arm, lean, braised	3 oz	184	7.1	0
shank cross cut, lean, simmered	3 oz	171	5.4	0
short rib, lean, braised	3 oz	251	15.4	0
Steak				
filet mignon, lean, broiled	3 oz	179	8.5	0
flank, lean, broiled	3 oz	176	8.6	0
porterhouse, lean, broiled	3 oz	185	9.2	0
rib eye, lean, broiled	3 oz	191	10	0
sirloin, wedge bone, lean, broiled	3 oz	166	6.1	0
T-bone, lean, broiled	3 oz	182	8.8	0
top round, lean, broiled	3 oz	153	4.2	0
Lamb				
Ground, broiled	3 oz	241	16.7	0
Kebab cubes, lean, broiled	3 oz	156	6.2	0
Leg, lean, roasted	3 oz	162	6.6	0
Rib roast, crown, lean, roasted	3 oz	197	11.3	0
Lunchmeats/Processed Meats				
Bologna				
beef	2 slices	177	16.2	0
turkey	2 slices	113	8.6	0
Bratwurst, fresh	1 link (3 oz)	256	22	0
Chicken roll, light meat	2 slices	90	4.2	0
Corned beef	2 slices	142	8.5	0
Frankfurter				
beef	1	180	16.3	0
chicken	1	116	8.8	0
Ham, boiled, extra-lean	2 slices	74	2.8	0
Kielbasa, smoked	2 slices (2 oz total)	176	15.4	0

FOOD	PORTION	CAL.	FAT (G)	FIBER (G)
Knockwurst, smoked	1 link (2½ oz)	209	18.9	0
Liverwurst, fresh	3 slices	185	16.2	0
Olive loaf, pork	2 slices	133	9.4	0
Pastrami				
beef	2 slices	198	16.6	0
turkey	2 slices	80	3.5	0
Pepperoni	10 slices	273	24.2	0
Pork sausage, fresh	4 links (2 oz total)	192	16.2	0
Salami, pork	3 slices	230	19.1	0
Scrapple	2 oz	120	7.6	0
Turkey breast	2 slices	47	0.7	0
Turkey ham	2 slices (2 oz total)	73	2.8	0
Pork				
Bacon				
Canadian	2 medium slices	86	3.9	0
smoked	3 medium slices	109	9.4	0
smoked, thickly sliced	1 slice	50	4.5	0
Chop, center rib, lean, roasted	3 oz	208	11.7	0
Ham, cured, roasted	3 oz	140	6.5	0
Roast, center loin, lean, roasted	3 oz	204	11.1	0
Spareribs, lean, braised	3 oz	337	25.8	0
Veal				
Ground, broiled	3 oz	146	6.4	0
Loin, lean, roasted	3 oz	149	5.9	0

MILK AND MILK PRODUCTS

FOOD	PORTION	CAL.	FAT (G)	FIBER (G)
Cream				
Half-and-half	2 Tbsp	39	3.5	0
Heavy	2 Tbsp	103	11	0

(continued)

MILK AND MILK PRODUCTS (CONT.)				
FOOD	**PORTION**	**CAL.**	**FAT (G)**	**FIBER (G)**
Cream (cont.)				
Light	2 Tbsp	59	5.8	0
Nondairy, powdered	1 tsp	10	0.5	0
flavored	1 tsp	60	3	0
Sour cream				
fat-free	2 Tbsp	30	0	0
reduced-fat	2 Tbsp	35	2	0
regular	2 Tbsp	62	6	0
Whipped cream	2 Tbsp	19	1.7	0
Whipped topping, nondairy	2 Tbsp	30	2.4	0
Milk				
1%	1 cup	102	2.6	0
1% chocolate	1 cup	158	2.5	1.2
2%	1 cup	121	4.7	0
Buttermilk	1 cup	99	2.2	0
Dairy shake mix, chocolate, prepared with water	6 oz	80	1	0
Dry, nonfat, prepared	1 cup	82	0.2	0
Eggnog	½ cup	171	9.5	0
Evaporated				
fat-free	2 Tbsp	25	0	0
regular	2 Tbsp	40	2	0
Fat-free	1 cup	86	0.4	0
Whole	1 cup	157	8.9	0
Whole, chocolate	1 cup	208	8.5	2
Yogurt				
Fruit, light	1 cup	100	0	0.4
Plain				
fat-free	1 cup	120	0	0
low-fat (1½% milk-fat)	1 cup	150	4	0
whole-milk	1 cup	139	7.4	0

NUTS AND SEEDS				
FOOD	**PORTION**	**CAL.**	**FAT (G)**	**FIBER (G)**
Nuts				
Almonds, unblanched, dried	1 oz	167	14.8	3.3
Brazil, unblanched, dried	1 oz	186	18.8	1.5
Cashews, dry-roasted	1 oz	163	13.2	0.9
Chestnuts, European, roasted	1 oz	70	0.6	3.7
Coconut, sweetened, flaked	1 oz	126	9	1.2
Filberts (hazelnuts), unblanched, dried	1 oz	179	17.8	2.8
Macadamia, dried	1 oz	199	20.9	2.3
Mixed, dry-roasted	1 oz	169	14.6	1.6
Peanuts, dry-roasted	1 oz	164	13.9	2.3
Pecans, dried	1 oz	189	19.2	2.6
Pine (pignolia), dried	1 oz	146	14.4	1.3
Pistachios, dried	1 oz	164	13.7	2.9
Walnuts, English, dried	1 oz	182	17.6	1.9
Seeds				
Pumpkin, dried, hulled	1 oz	154	13	1.1
Sesame, dried, hulled	1 Tbsp	47	4.4	0.9
Sunflower, dried	1 oz	162	14.1	3.3

PASTA				
FOOD	**PORTION**	**CAL.**	**FAT (G)**	**FIBER (G)**
Cooked Pasta				
Fresh	1 cup	183	1.5	0
Macaroni, enriched	1 cup	197	0.9	1.8
Noodles				
egg, enriched	1 cup	213	2.4	1.8
soba	1 cup	113	0.1	0
Spaghetti				
enriched	1 cup	197	0.9	2.4
whole wheat	1 cup	174	0.8	6.3
Spinach, fresh	1 cup	182	1.3	0
Tortellini	½ cup	220	5	0

(continued)

PASTA (CONT.)

FOOD	PORTION	CAL.	FAT (G)	FIBER (G)
Pasta Dishes				
Fettuccine Alfredo, frozen	9 oz	270	7	2
Macaroni and cheese, homemade, baked	1 cup	430	22.2	1
Manicotti, cheese, frozen	3 oz	290	9	4
Pasta primavera, frozen	10 oz	260	8	4
Pasta salad with seafood, without dressing	3½ oz	90	5	0
Ravioli, cheese, with tomato sauce, frozen	9½ oz	360	14	4
Spaghetti and meatballs, homemade	1 cup	332	11.7	8
Tortellini, cheese, with tomato sauce, frozen	9 oz	290	6	4

PIZZA

FOOD	PORTION	CAL.	FAT (G)	FIBER (G)
Cheese				
Chef Boyardee, dry mix, prepared	1 slice	320	8	2
Domino's thin crust	⅓ of 12" pie	364	15.5	1.9
Healthy Choice French bread pizza	1	310	4	6
Pizza Hut thin crust	1 slice of medium pie	205	8	2
Weight Watchers extra cheese	1	390	12	6
Italian sausage				
Domino's hand-tossed, with mushrooms	2 slices of 12" pie	402	13.9	3
Healthy Choice sausage French bread pizza	1	330	4	6
Pizza Hut hand-tossed	1 slice of medium pie	267	11	2
Pepperoni				
Domino's hand-tossed	2 slices of 12" pie	406	15.1	2

FOOD	PORTION	CAL.	FAT (G)	FIBER (G)
Healthy Choice pepperoni French bread pizza	1	350	9	5
Pizza Hut hand-tossed	1 slice of medium pie	238	8	2
Weight Watchers	1	390	12	4
Supreme				
Lean Cuisine deluxe French bread pizza	1	330	6	4
Pizza Hut hand-tossed	1 slice of medium pie	284	12	3
Weight Watchers deluxe combo	1	380	11	6
Veggie				
Domino's hand-tossed	2 slices of 12" pie	360	10.4	3
Pizza Hut hand-tossed	1 slice of medium pie	216	6	3

POULTRY, FOWL, AND GAME

FOOD	PORTION	CAL.	FAT (G)	FIBER (G)
Capon, roasted, without skin	3 oz	195	9.9	0
Chicken				
breast, without skin				
fried in batter	½ (3 oz)	161	4.1	0
roasted	½ (3 oz)	142	3.1	0
breast, with skin				
fried in batter	½ (5 oz)	364	18.5	0.2
roasted	½ (4 oz)	193	7.6	0
drumstick, with skin				
fried in batter	1 (3 oz)	193	11.3	0.2
roasted	1 (2 oz)	112	5.8	0
liver, simmered	3 oz	133	4.6	0
thigh, without skin				
fried in batter	1 (2 oz)	113	5.4	0.2
roasted	1 (2 oz)	109	5.7	0

(continued)

POULTRY, FOWL, AND GAME (CONT.)

FOOD	PORTION	CAL.	FAT (G)	FIBER (G)
Duck, roasted, without skin	3 oz	171	9.5	0
Pâté				
chicken, canned	1 oz	57	3.7	0
goose, smoked, canned	1 oz	131	12.4	0
Pheasant, meat only, uncooked	3 oz	113	3.1	0
Potpie, chicken, homemade	1 piece (8 oz)	550	31.3	3
Rabbit, roasted	3 oz	131	5.4	0
Squab (pigeon), uncooked	1 (6 oz)	239	12.6	0
Turkey				
breast, prebasted, roasted, without skin	3 oz	107	2.9	0
dark meat, roasted, without skin	3 oz	32	1.2	0
dark meat, roasted, with skin	3 oz	188	9.8	0
light meat, roasted, without skin	3 oz	34	0.7	0
light meat, roasted, with skin	3 oz	168	7.1	0
liver, simmered	3 oz	144	5.1	0
Venison, roasted	3 oz	134	2.7	0

SOUPS AND STEWS

FOOD	PORTION	CAL.	FAT (G)	FIBER (G)
Soups				
Beef noodle, condensed, made with water	1 cup	83	3.1	0.7
Beef vegetable, condensed, made with water	1 cup	78	1.9	0.5
Black bean, condensed, made with water	1 cup	116	1.5	1.4
Bouillon, beef, from cube, made with water	1 cup	7	0.2	0
Bouillon, chicken, from cube, made with water	1 cup	12	0.3	0

FOOD	PORTION	CAL.	FAT (G)	FIBER (G)
Cheese, condensed, made with water	1 cup	156	10.5	1
Chicken noodle, condensed, made with water	1 cup	75	2.5	0.7
Chicken rice, condensed, made with water	1 cup	60	1.9	1
Clam chowder				
Manhattan, condensed, made with water	1 cup	78	2.2	3.5
New England, low-fat	1 cup	120	2	1
Crab, canned, ready-to-serve	1 cup	76	1.5	0.7
Cream of celery, condensed, made with water	1 cup	90	5.6	0.7
Cream of chicken, condensed, made with water	1 cup	117	7.4	0.2
Cream of mushroom, condensed, made with water	1 cup	129	9	0.5
Cream of potato, condensed, made with water	1 cup	73	2.4	0.5
Gazpacho, canned, ready-to-serve	1 cup	46	2.2	0.5
Green pea, condensed, made with water	1 cup	165	2.9	2.6
Lentil with ham	1 cup	139	2.8	1
Minestrone	1 cup	204	5	2
Onion, condensed, made with water	1 cup	58	1.7	1
Scotch broth, condensed, made with water	1 cup	80	2.6	1.2
Split pea with ham, low-fat	1 cup	170	2.5	2
Tomato, condensed, made with water	½ cup	100	2	0.5
Turkey vegetable, condensed, made with water	1 cup	72	3	0.5
Vegetarian vegetable, condensed, made with water	1 cup	72	1.9	0.5

(continued)

SOUPS AND STEWS (CONT.)				
FOOD	**PORTION**	**CAL.**	**FAT (G)**	**FIBER (G)**
Stews				
Beef, ready-to-serve	1 cup	194	7.6	3.4
Oyster, condensed, made with water	1 cup	58	3.8	0

VEGETABLES				
FOOD	**PORTION**	**CAL.**	**FAT (G)**	**FIBER (G)**
Broccoli, boiled	½ cup	22	0.3	2.3
Cabbage, boiled, shredded	½ cup	17	0.3	2.1
Carrot, raw	1	31	0.1	2.1
Chile peppers, raw, chopped	½ cup	30	0.2	1.1
Corn, sweet yellow, boiled	Kernels from 1 ear	83	1	2.2
Eggplant, boiled, cubed	½ cup	13	0.1	1.2
Garlic, raw	1 clove	4	0.02	0.1
Okra, boiled	½ cup	26	0.1	2
Onions, raw, chopped	½ cup	30	0.1	1.4
Potatoes				
Au gratin	½ cup	161	9.2	2.2
Baked				
plain, flesh only	1 (6 oz)	145	0.2	2.3
plain, microwaved, flesh and skin	1 (8 oz)	212	0.2	2.3
with sour cream and chives	1 (6 oz)	221	12.6	5
Boiled, flesh only	1	67	0.1	1.4
French fries				
deep-fried	20–25 1"–2" strips	235	12.2	2
frozen, oven-heated	20 (4 oz total)	222	8.8	3.2
microwave	1 box (3 oz)	230	12	2
Mashed, made with whole milk and margarine	½ cup	111	4.4	2.1
Potato pancake	1 (3 oz)	234	12.6	1.5

FOOD	PORTION	CAL.	FAT (G)	FIBER (G)
Potato salad	½ cup	179	10.3	3.3
Scalloped	½ cup	105	4.5	2.3
Sweet potato, baked	1 (4 oz)	117	0.1	3.4
Pumpkin, canned	½ cup	41	0.3	3.4
Tomatoes, raw, chopped	1 cup	38	0.6	2.0
Zucchini, raw, sliced	½ cup	9	0.1	0.8

CALORIE BURN FOR 250 EXERCISES AND COMMON ACTIVITIES

Not only is exercise crucial to weight loss, but breaking a sweat on a regular basis may also help you keep those pounds off. The government guideline: moderate exercise for 30 to 45 minutes, 3 to 5 days a week.

As you decide what type of exercise to do, keep in mind that different activities burn vastly different amounts of calories. Here's how to find the calorie burn for your favorite exercise.

The first thing you need to know is your weight in kilograms. One kilogram equals 2.2 pounds, but rather than doing the math to find your weight equivalent, simply use the chart below. First, find your weight in pounds in the left-hand column, then check the right-hand column for the kilogram equivalent. A 150-pound woman, for example, weighs 68 kilograms.

POUNDS	KILOGRAMS
95	43
100	45
105	48
110	50
115	52
120	55

POUNDS	KILOGRAMS
125	57
130	59
135	61
140	64
145	66
150	68

POUNDS	KILOGRAMS
155	70
160	73
165	75
170	77
175	80
180	82
185	84
190	86
195	89
200	91
205	93
210	95

POUNDS	KILOGRAMS
215	98
220	100
225	102
230	105
235	107
240	109
245	111
250	114
255	116
260	118
265	120
270	123

The second factor in the formula is the MET (metabolic equivalent) value, which is an expression of the rate of energy expenditure for physical activity. One MET is the energy expended by an average adult at rest, which equals about 1 calorie burned per kilogram of body weight per hour. Thus, the energy expenditure for a 60-kilogram person sitting quietly is approximately 60 calories per hour.

To find your calorie burn per hour for a specific activity, find the exercise in the following chart, then multiply its MET value by your weight in kilograms. For example, if you weigh 68 kilograms and you want to see how many calories you burn on a 12 mph leisurely 1-hour bike ride, multiply the MET value of 8 by your body weight of 68. That gives you 544 calories burned per hour. If you're exercising for a half-hour, multiply the hourly rate by 0.5 (= 272 calories burned); for 15 minutes, multiply by 0.25 (= 136 calories burned).

Here's a list of 250 common activities and their MET values.

EXERCISE	MET
Bicycling	
<10 mph, leisure, to work, for pleasure	4
10–11.9 mph, leisure, slow, light effort	6
12–13.9 mph, leisure, moderate effort	8
14–15.9 mph, racing or leisure, fast, vigorous effort	10
16–19 mph, racing/not drafting or not more than 19 mph drafting, very fast, racing	12
BMX, mountain biking	8.5
Unicycling	5
Conditioning Exercises	
Aerobics, high-impact	7
Aerobics, low-impact	5
Aerobics, step, 6–8" step	8.5
Aerobics, teaching class	6
Bicycling, stationary, general	7
Calisthenics (push-ups, sit-ups, pull-ups, jumping jacks), heavy, vigorous effort	8
Circuit training, some aerobic movement with minimal rest	8
Rowing machine	7
Ski machine	7
Stairclimber or treadmill	9
Stretching, hatha yoga	2.5
Weight lifting (free weights; Nautilus or Universal-type), light or moderate effort, light workout	3
Dancing	
Ballet or modern, twist, jazz, tap, jitterbug	4.8
Ballroom, fast (disco, folk, square), line dancing, Irish step dancing, polka, contra, country	4.5
Ballroom, slow (waltz, fox-trot, slow dancing), samba, tango, mambo, cha-cha	3
General, Greek, Middle Eastern, hula, flamenco, belly dancing, swing	4.5

EXERCISE	MET
Fishing and Hunting	
Fishing, from boat, sitting	2.5
Fishing, from riverbank, walking	4
Hunting, duck, wading	2.5
Hunting, general	5
Hunting, pheasant or grouse	6
Hunting, rabbit, squirrel, prairie chick, raccoon, or small game	5
Pistol or trap shooting, standing	2.5
Household Activities	
Caregiving, elderly or disabled adult, active periods only	4
Carpentry, finishing or refinishing cabinets or furniture	4.5
Carrying groceries up stairs	7.5
Carrying small child	3
Cleaning, heavy or major (washing car, washing windows, cleaning garage), vigorous effort	3
Cleaning gutters	5
Cooking or food preparation, standing or sitting, manual appliances	2
Cooking or food preparation, walking or standing, serving food, setting table	2.5
Eating, sitting	1.5
Grooming, personal (washing, shaving, brushing teeth, washing hands, applying makeup), sitting or standing	2
Ironing	2.3
Mopping floor	3.5
Multiple household tasks, simultaneous, light effort	2.5
Multiple household tasks, simultaneous, moderate effort	3.5
Painting, papering, plastering, scraping, hanging Sheetrock, remodeling indoors	3
Putting away groceries, carrying groceries or packages	2.5
Repairing car	3
Scrubbing floors, on hands and knees, scrubbing bathroom	3.8

(continued)

EXERCISE	MET
Household Activities (cont.)	
Shopping, food, with or without a cart, standing or walking	2.3
Shopping, general, standing or walking	2.3
Standing, bathing dog	3.5
Standing, light (pumping gas, changing lightbulb, etc.)	2
Standing, playing with children, light, active periods only	2.8
Sweeping garage, sidewalk, or outside of house	4
Vacuuming	3.5
Walking/running, playing with animals, moderate, active periods only	4
Walking/running, playing with children, moderate, active periods only	4
Washing and waxing car, hull of boat, airplane	4.5
Washing dishes, standing and walking	2.5
Watering plants	2.5
Lawn Care and Gardening	
Carrying, loading, stacking wood, loading/unloading, carrying lumber	5
Digging, spading, filling in garden, composting	5
Mowing lawn, power mower, walking	5.5
Mowing lawn, riding mower	2.5
Operating snow blower, walking	4.5
Planting seedlings, shrubs	4.5
Raking lawn	4.3
Shoveling snow, by hand	6
Trimming shrubs, trees, manual trimmer	4.5
Trimming shrubs, trees, power trimmer, using leaf blower, edger	3.5
Walking, standing, cleaning up yard, light, picking flowers or vegetables	4
Watering lawn, garden, standing or walking	1.5
Weeding, cultivating garden	4.5

EXERCISE	MET
Musical Performance	
Accordion	1.8
Cello	2
Conducting, band or orchestra	2.5
Drums	4
Flute	2
Guitar, classical, folk, sitting	2
Guitar, rock band, standing	3
Horn	2
Marching in band, playing instrument, twirling baton	4
Piano/organ	2.5
Trombone	3.5
Trumpet	2.5
Violin	2.5
Woodwind	2
Occupational Activities	
Construction, outdoors, remodeling	2.5
Driving truck, loading/unloading, standing	6.5
Farming, animal care (grooming, brushing, shearing, medical care)	6
Farming, baling hay, forking straw bales, cleaning corral, barn, poultry work, vigorous effort	8
Fire fighting	12
Giving professional massage, standing	4
Sitting, in meetings, general, talking, eating at business meeting	1.5
Sitting, light office work, general (chemistry lab work, light use of hand tools, watch repair, microassembly, light assembly/repair), sitting, reading, driving	1.5
Skin/scuba diving, as frogman (Navy Seal)	12
Standing, light/moderate (heavy assembly/repair, welding, stocking, auto repair, packing moving boxes), patient care (nursing)	3

(continued)

EXERCISE	MET
Occupational Activities (cont.)	
Tailoring, hand sewing	2
Tailoring, machine sewing	2.5
Teaching physical education, exercise, sports classes	6.5
Typing, electric, manual, computer	1.5
Using heavy power tools, jackhammer, drill	6
Quiet and Light Activities	
Lying quietly watching television, doing nothing, lying in bed awake, listening to music (not talking or reading)	1
Meditating	1
Reclining, talking, talking on phone, reading	1
Sitting, reading book, newspaper	1.3
Sitting, studying (reading and/or writing, desk work, typing), in class (note-taking or class discussion)	1.8
Sitting, talking, talking on the phone, playing cards or board games, sitting at a sporting event	1.5
Sitting, watching television, smoking, listening to music (not talking or reading), watching a movie in a theater	1
Sleeping	0.9
Standing, arts and crafts, light effort	1.8
Standing quietly (waiting in line)	1.2
Standing, reading, talking, talking on the phone	1.8
Running	
5 mph (12 min./mile)	8
6 mph (10 min./mile)	10
7.5 mph (8 min./mile)	12.5
10 mph (6 min./mile)	16
Jogging, in place	8
Jogging, on mini-trampoline	4.5
Up stairs	15

EXERCISE	MET
Sexual Activity	
Active, vigorous effort	1.5
General, moderate effort	1.3
Passive, light effort, kissing, hugging	1
Sports	
Archery, nonhunting	3.5
Badminton, social singles and doubles, general	4.5
Baseball, playing catch	2.5
Baseball, softball, fast or slow pitch, general	5
Basketball, casual, general	6
Basketball, shooting baskets	4.5
Basketball, wheelchair	6.5
Billiards	2.5
Bowling	3
Boxing, punching bag	6
Boxing, sparring	9
Broomball	7
Children's games, hopscotch, 4-square, dodgeball, playground apparatus, T-ball, tetherball, marbles, jacks, arcade games	5
Coaching, football, soccer, basketball, baseball, swimming	4
Cricket, batting, bowling	5
Croquet	2.5
Curling	4
Darts, wall, lawn	2.5
Fencing	6
Football, competitive	9
Football, touch, flag, general	8
Frisbee	3
Golf, miniature, driving range	3
Golf, using power cart	3.5

(continued)

EXERCISE	MET
Sports (cont.)	
Golf, walking and carrying clubs	4.5
Golf, walking and pulling clubs	4.3
Gymnastics	4
Hacky Sack	4
Handball, general	12
Handball, team	8
Hockey, field, ice	8
Horseback riding, trotting	6.5
Horseback riding, walking	2.5
Horseshoes, quoits	3
Jai alai	12
Judo, jujitsu	10
Juggling	4
Karate, tae kwan do	10
Kickball	7
Kickboxing	10
Lacrosse	8
Orienteering	9
Paddleball, casual	6
Polo	9
Racquetball, casual	7
Racquetball, competitive	10
Rock climbing, ascending	11
Rock climbing, rappelling	8
Rope jumping, fast	12
Rope jumping, moderate	10
Rope jumping, slow	8
Rugby	10

EXERCISE	MET
Shuffleboard, lawn bowling	3
Skateboarding	5
Skating, in-line	12
Skating, roller	7
Soccer, competitive	10
Soccer, casual, general	7
Squash	12
Table tennis, Ping-Pong	4
Tai chi	4
Tennis, doubles	5
Tennis, singles	8
Track and field, high jump, long jump, triple jump, javelin, pole vault	6
Track and field, shot put, discus, hammer	4
Track and field, steeplechase, hurdles	10
Trampoline	3.5
Volleyball, casual, 6–9-member team	3
Volleyball, competitive, indoor, beach	8
Wallyball	7
Wrestling (5-min. match)	6
Travel and Transportation	
Driving heavy truck, tractor, bus	3
Riding in car, truck	1
Riding motor scooter, motorcycle	2.5
Touring/traveling/vacation, walking and riding	2
Walking	
Less than 2 mph, level surface, strolling, very slow	2
2 mph, firm level surface, slow	2.5
2.5 mph, firm surface, walking dog	3
2.5 mph, downhill	2.8

(continued)

EXERCISE	MET
Walking (cont.)	
3 mph, firm level surface, moderate	3.3
3 mph, moderate, carrying objects less than 25 lb.	4
3.5 mph, firm level surface, brisk, walking for exercise	3.8
3.5 mph, uphill	6
4 mph, firm level surface, very brisk	5
4.5 mph, firm level surface, extremely brisk	6.3
Bird watching	2.5
Climbing hills, 0- to 9-lb. load	7
Climbing hills, 10- to 20-lb. load	7.5
Climbing hills, 21- to 42-lb. load	8
Climbing hills, 42+ lb. load	9
Going down stairs, standing, carrying objects 25–49 lb.	5
Hiking, cross-country	6
Pushing wheelchair	4
Racewalking	6.5
Using crutches	5
With children, pushing or pulling child in stroller	2.5
Water Activities	
Canoeing, on camping trip	4
Canoeing, rowing, competitive, crew or sculling	12
Canoeing, rowing, for pleasure	3.5
Diving, springboard or platform	3
Kayaking	5
Rafting, kayaking, canoeing, whitewater	5
Sailing, ocean, yachting	3
Sailing, Sunfish/Laser/Hobie Cat, keel boat	3
Skin diving, moderate	12.5
Skin/scuba diving, general	7

EXERCISE	MET
Snorkeling	5
Surfing, body or board	3
Swimming, breaststroke, general	10
Swimming, butterfly, general	11
Swimming, crawl, slow (50 yd./min.), moderate or light effort	8
Swimming, laps, freestyle, fast, vigorous effort	10
Swimming, laps, freestyle, slow, moderate or light effort	7
Swimming, leisurely, not laps, general	6
Swimming, synchronized	8
Water aerobics/calisthenics	4
Water jogging	8
Water polo	10
Waterskiing	6
Winter Activities	
Skating, ice, 9 mph or less	5.5
Skiing, cross-country, 2.5 mph, slow or light effort, ski walking	7
Skiing, cross-country, 4 to 4.9 mph, moderate speed and effort, general	8
Skiing, downhill, moderate effort, general	6
Skiing, downhill, vigorous effort, racing	8
Sledding, tobogganing, bobsledding, luge	7
Snowmobiling	3.5
Snowshoeing	8

SOURCE: Printed with permission from Barbara Ainsworth, Ph.D., of the exercise science department at the University of South Carolina in Columbia.

ABOUT THE AUTHORS

CATHY NONAS, M.S., R.D., C.D.E., is director of the VanItallie Center for Nutrition and Weight Management, an arm of the New York Obesity Research Center at St. Luke's–Roosevelt Hospital Center in New York City. The Obesity Research Center is one of four federally funded centers for investigating the causes and treatment of obesity in the United States.

JENNIFER BRIGHT has researched, written, and edited health publications for more than 5 years, including the books *Seniors Guide to Pain-Free Living* and *The Immune Advantage*.

JULIA VANTINE is a health journalist whose most recent books include *Maximum Food Power for Women* and *Energy for Everything: Rejuvenation for the Mind, Body, and Soul.*

To purchase
another copy of the

OUTWIT YOUR WEIGHT JOURNAL

or a copy of the book

OUTWIT YOUR WEIGHT,

visit your local bookstore,
call (800) 848-4735, or visit

www.rodalestore.com

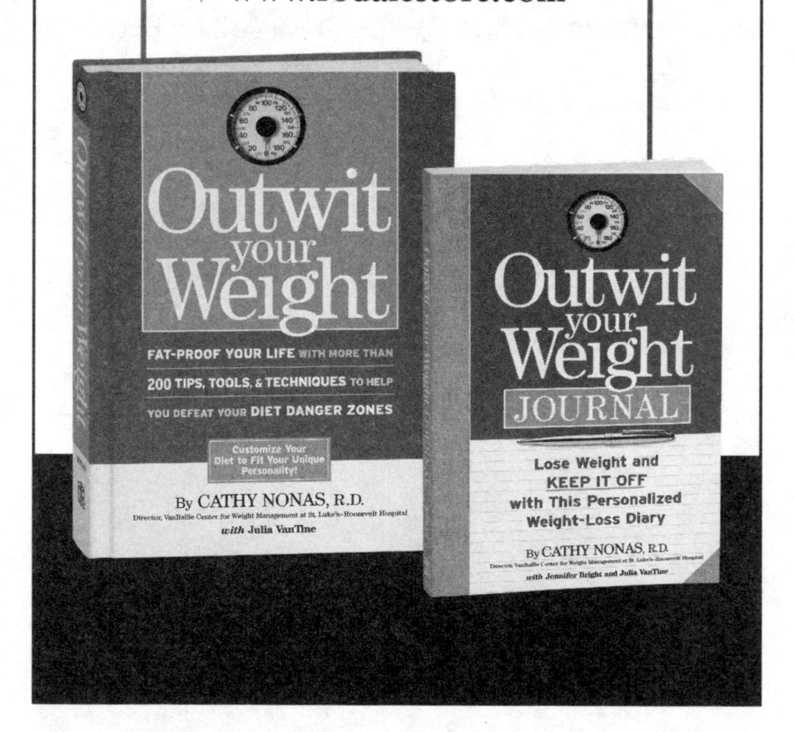